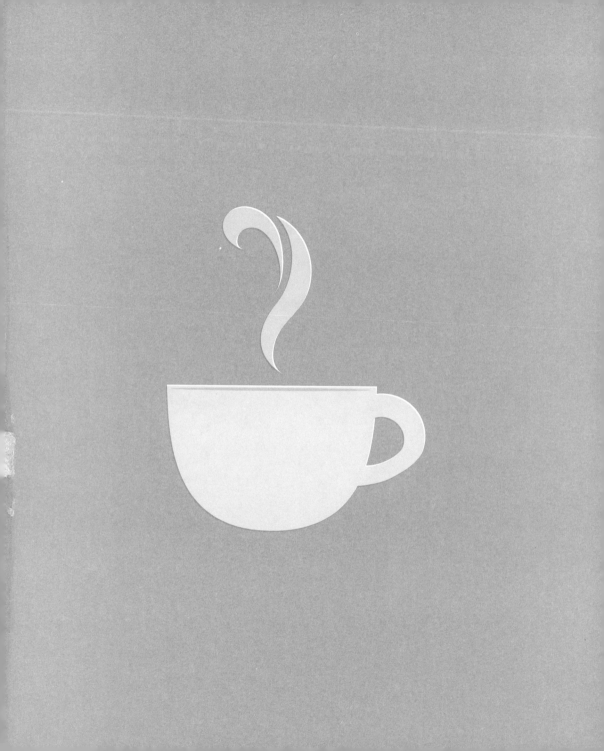

THE COFFEE LOVER'S DIET

WILLIAM MORROW
An Imprint of HarperCollinsPublishers

THE COFFEE LOVER'S DIET

CHANGE YOUR COFFEE, CHANGE YOUR LIFE

BOB ARNOT, M.D.

Data in "Top Ten Sources of Antioxidants in U.S. Diet" chart in chapter 1 courtesy of Joe Vinson, Ph.D., University of Scranton, Pennsylvania.

Data in "Depression Risk Reduction" chart in chapter 1 from Michel Lucas, Ph.D., R.D., et al., "Coffee, Caffeine, and Risk of Depression Among Women," *Archives of Internal Medicine* 171, no. 17 (September 26, 2011): 1571–78.

"Flavor Emphasis by Roast Degree" chart in chapter 3 re-created with permission from Coffee Analysts of Hinesburg, Vermont.

"SCAA Grind Description" table in chapter 4 re-created with permission from SCAA.

"SCAA Ideal Water Characteristics" table in chapter 4 re-created with permission from SCAA.

Data in "High-Phenol Foods" chart in chapter 5 courtesy of the Phenol-Expolorer database.

This book contains advice and information relating to health care. It should be used to supplement rather than replace the advice of your doctor or another trained health professional. If you know or suspect you have a health problem, it is recommended that you seek your physician's advice before embarking on any medical program or treatment. All efforts have been made to assure the accuracy of the information contained in this book as of the date of publication. This publisher and the author disclaim liability for any medical outcomes that may occur as a result of applying the methods suggested in this book.

HarperCollins books may be purchased for educational, business, or sales promotional use. For information please e-mail the Special Markets Department at SPsales@harpercollins.com.

FIRST EDITION

DESIGNED BY WILLIAM RUOTO

Library of Congress Cataloging-in-Publication Data has been applied for.

ISBN 978-0-06-245877-3

17 18 19 20 21   LSC   10 9 8 7 6 5 4 3 2 1

LIFE IS MADE WORTHWHILE BY THOSE WITH WHOM

WE TAKE THE JOURNEY. I'D LIKE TO DEDICATE

THIS BOOK TO THOSE WHO HAVE MADE MINE

SO WONDERFUL AND INSPIRED: FIRST, TO MY

THREE WONDERFUL SONS, BOBBY, HAYDEN,

AND ALYSDAIR, WHO BRING BRIGHTNESS INTO

EVERY DAY; SECOND, TO MY LOVELY BROTHERS

AND SISTERS, BONNIE, DOUGIE, JEANNE, PAUL,

AND NANCY, WHO HAVE MADE SO MUCH OF THIS

JOURNEY WITH ME; FINALLY, TO MY FIANCÉE,

AMY STEWART, WHO INSPIRED ME TO BECOME A

COFFEE ENTHUSIAST AND TO WRITE THIS BOOK.

CONTENTS

PART III THE COFFEE LOVER'S DIET

Early one morning a few years ago, I joined a dozen riders outside the house of a cycling coach named David Kinjah, in a small village outside of Kikuyu, Kenya. The look of our skintight Lycra and the latest in bicycle technology contrasted sharply with the rustic housing. Around me stood Kenya's top cycling team, Safari Simbaz. They were lean and impossibly fit, and I was going to ride with them. We set off a short while later from the city center, where the roads were rough, pocked with potholes, and massed with traffic, including giant transport trucks that belched smoke into the air. We emerged from the chaos onto spectacular, newly paved roads in a landscape of emerald-green fields, and began the climb into the mountains. As the elevation rose toward seven thousand feet, I was gasping for air, struggling to keep up with Africa's best.

After a series of arduous ascents and terrifying descents, finally, we pulled over at a small roadside restaurant. The little place served only locally produced fare, and the team emphasized how clean foods improve their performance. In the tiny kitchen I spied some coffee beans and picked one up. Holding it up in the sunlight, I saw that it was wonderfully light in color. We sat down side by side on benches as the beans were ground and brewed. Then the coffee came. It was a brew like I had never experienced. I'd never known that coffee had such flavors, but they hit my palate like those of the finest French wine: Concord grapes, fresh-cut cedar, sweet grapefruit, and red currants. The coffee had a bright acidity, with a full, juicy, syrupy body. My brain came to life with concentration and attention that cut through the early morning grogginess. Back on the road, my legs had renewed power and drive. I soared up the hills, hanging on to the pack and marveling at the power and purity of Kenyan coffee. It's little wonder the nation has some of the world's best endurance athletes with coffee like this!

I'm fortunate to have had a long career as a physician, journalist, and author. I'm also an athlete, a humanitarian, and a science buff. In recent years, I've grown passionate about coffee because it appeals to me on all of these fronts. Coffee is the new red wine. There are tasting courses, sommeliers, and aficionados tracking single-origin beans from remote estates and terroirs around the globe. Coffee contains twelve hundred flavor compounds to red wine's seven hundred. Amazing. But did you know that coffee is also the new weapon in weight loss? The new sports drink? The highest source of antioxidants in the American diet? Perhaps, even, the most cost-effective prevention for many fatal diseases?

ABOLISHING DOUBT

I've written more than a dozen books on nutrition. When I was chief medical correspondent for *Dateline NBC, Today, NBC Nightly News,* and *CBS Evening News* from the 1980s into the 2000s, I was always on the lookout for the next great nutrition story. Ironically, I was particularly alert to stories about why coffee was bad for you. At that time, coffee had a reputation for causing harm, and most people feared that it was unhealthy. Why? Early studies weren't sophisticated enough, nor were they large enough to tease out specific variables. Since coffee drinking often occurred in tandem with poor health markers such as smoking, diets bereft of fruits and vegetables, sedentary lifestyles, and even obesity, the assumption was that coffee caused similar poor outcomes.

So I was stunned when, in 2012, I read the results of an enormous study undertaken by the prestigious National Institutes of Health, announcing that "older adults who drank coffee—caffeinated or decaffeinated—had a lower risk of death overall than others who did not drink coffee."[1] Coffee drinkers were less likely to die from heart disease, respiratory disease, stroke, injuries and accidents, diabetes, and infections, the study concluded. The more coffee people drank, the better they fared. Coffee appeared to be the superfood of all superfoods. The more I learned, the more I wanted to know.

Soon the venerable *New England Journal of Medicine* published a comprehensive study using data from the NIH. Their analysis, involving four hundred thousand participants, found that significant coffee consumption reduced the risk of death from all causes by 15 percent in women and by 10 percent in men.[2]

As evidence of coffee's robust, positive effect on health piled up, the main scientific advisory arm of the U.S. government published a spectacular report in 2015. Part of the new U.S. dietary guidelines, the report launched a sea change in public appreciation of coffee.

> Currently, strong evidence shows that consumption of coffee within the moderate range (3 to 5 cups per day or up to 400 milligrams per day of caffeine) is not associated with increased long-term health risks among healthy individuals. In fact, consistent evidence indicates that coffee consumption is associated with reduced risk of type 2 diabetes and cardiovascular disease in adults. Moreover, moderate evidence shows a protective association between caffeine intake and risk of Parkinson's

BOB ARNOT, M.D.

disease. Therefore, moderate coffee consumption can be incorporated into a healthy dietary pattern, along with other healthful behaviors.

—2015 U.S. Dietary Guidelines Advisory Committee[3]

In October 2016 came yet another clincher, this time from the *European Journal of Epidemiology*. A review of thirty-one studies and 1,610,543 individuals confirmed the staggering decreased risk for coffee drinkers in all causes of death, including cardiovascular disease and cancer.[4]

PARADISE

Meanwhile, National Geographic Fellow Dan Buettner was gathering information about groups of people who are living longer, healthier lives than anyone else on Earth. They live in five geographic areas known as Blue Zones. Distributed across the globe, these populations outlive Americans by roughly a decade. The Blue Zones are

OKINAWA, JAPAN

SARDINIA, ITALY

NICOYA PENINSULA, COSTA RICA

LOMA LINDA, CALIFORNIA, UNITED STATES

IKARIA, GREECE

That last one particularly interested me. Every acre of the idyllic island of Ikaria, set in the blue-green Aegean sea, drips with beauty and charm. In a 2012 *New York Times Magazine* article, Dan Buettner called Ikaria "the island where people forget to die."

The island earned this title because one in three Ikarians lives into their nineties. Still physically active in their later years, Ikarians reach age ninety at two and a half times the rate Americans do. (Ikarian men are nearly four times as likely to reach age ninety as American men.) Not only are they living roughly ten years longer than most of us in the United States or Europe, older Ikarians maintain active sex lives. They suffer lower rates of depression, dementia, heart disease, and cancer.

Researchers have studied what makes the Ikarians so successful at living well and aging slowly. They walk the steeply pitched streets that are carved into their mountainous countryside. Villagers enjoy low stress and deep social networks. Their Mediterranean diet includes olive oil, red wine, fish, herbal tea, honey, potatoes, black-eyed peas, lentils, and limited amounts of meat, sugar, and dairy. Rich in beans and greens, their diet is loaded with antioxidants. Rare are the refined sugars and red meat that pervade the Western diet. And, my favorite, they nap!

We've heard much of this story before, however, of people who outlive us by decades. What's really unique about the Ikarians? Their coffee.

A team of Athens-based researchers discovered that Greek coffee contributes to the incredible good health of the Ikarians. The researchers found that 87 percent of their study participants drank boiled Greek coffee every day. The key finding was this: The more Greek coffee the Ikarians drank, the better their vascular health was. Vascular health (a layman's term for endothelial cell function) indicates the suppleness of blood vessels and their ability to respond to stress. We have sixty thousand miles of blood vessels coursing through our bodies, nourishing every organ we have. If our arteries remain young and supple, so will we. The Ikarian study found a previously undiscovered, direct link between coffee drinking and improved vascular health.[5]

CHANGE YOUR COFFEE, CHANGE YOUR LIFE

The new research leaves no room for doubt: Drinking coffee can be the healthiest indulgence of your day. Coffee can sharpen your focus, jump-start your workout, boost your performance, help you achieve sustained weight loss, and even fend off many causes of death. However, most coffee drinkers are missing out on the incredible benefits that coffee can provide. The coffee concoctions that many people drink are nutritional nightmares, packed with devastating amounts of fat and sugar. Even many black coffees are made from low-quality, overroasted beans that offer few health benefits. The way that Ikarians experience coffee is a far cry from the way most Americans consume it. We aren't reaping the full rewards of coffee, because the coffees we favor have lost their healthy components as well as their flavor, so we load them with cream and sugar and syrups that make us fat.

This book will teach you to leave the bad things behind and get the most good out of coffee. Two substances provide its primary benefits: caffeine and polyphenols, which are the same compounds that make fresh fruits and vegetables, red wines, and teas healthy. Polyphenols exert powerful antioxidant and anti-inflammatory effects on the body, fighting the forces that fuel many diseases. They provide many of coffee's health benefits. Happily for those who can't handle much caffeine, phenols, as we'll call them in this book, are present in decaffeinated coffee as well. In a cup of regular, they even have the power to blunt the jittery effect of caffeine, delivering smoother energy and focus. One of the most important concepts to take from this book is the knowledge that some coffee beans contain far more phenols than others. Those that are packed with the highest levels of these anti-inflammatory antioxidant compounds I like to call high-phenol coffees.

In the coming chapters you'll learn how to identify high-phenol coffees, which roasts to look for, and how best to grind and brew your coffee. We'll teach you to make coffee

BOB ARNOT, M.D.

so delicious you wouldn't dream of polluting it with sugar or half-and-half. Whether you need to lose weight, whether you're a foodie looking to enhance your sensory experiences or a black-coffee performance athlete, this book will help you choose the right coffee and vastly improve your enjoyment of it. You'll learn to sidestep the pitfalls of your current coffee habit to discover, instead, the perks of the world's best coffees. This book is your key to unlocking their amazing potential.

GREEK COFFEE

Excited about the power of a drink that so many people already love, I took a closer look at how the Greek coffee enjoyed by people living in the Blue Zone of Ikaria could deliver such spectacular results.

The most unique aspect of Greek coffee (in truth it's Turkish coffee, but Greeks can't bear to call it that) is the size of the grind. Greek coffee is literally a powder. Scientific literature on coffee shows that the finer the grind, the more surface area is opened up for extraction of the core ingredients in coffee, including phenols, caffeine, fats, flavor, and aroma. A coarsely ground bean yields 384 particles, while the powdery Greek grind yields nearly five hundred thousand particles from one bean.

Another notable feature of Greek coffee is the boiling water temperature. Like fine grinds, higher water temperatures also produce better extraction from coffee beans, according to the Specialty Coffee Association of America (SCAA). A scientific research paper[6] that compared all the common techniques for brewing coffee showed that boiling ranked number one in extracting the most important of all phenols: chlorogenic acid.

Finally, Ikarians skip a filter. An elegant study from Denmark[7] shows that cafestol, a key fat extracted by boiling coffee, helps the body make more insulin and use it better. While ordinary filtered coffee contains 0.1 milligrams of cafestol, unfiltered boiled coffee has 6–12 milligrams per cup. Consuming large amounts of cafestol, like any fat, can ultimately raise cholesterol, but moderate amounts of it, combined with high levels of phenols, appear to give Greek coffee its stunning health value—and the incredible ability to help muscles clear sugar from the bloodstream.

THE COFFEE LOVER'S DIET

The news from the idyllic island of Ikaria, from the NIH, from *The New England Journal of Medicine,* and from so many other sources kept percolating in my brain, ultimately compelling me to set off on an ambitious quest. I spent more than

BOB ARNOT, M.D.

a year searching the globe for the healthiest, most delicious coffees I could find. This book will take you along the trail I set, seeking the very best of beans, but also roasts, grinds, and brewing techniques, and putting them to the test. I took the highest-quality coffee beans to leading analytical chemistry facilities for months of testing. Since phenols supply many of coffee's health benefits, determining phenol content seemed a critical step that almost no one had taken. As a physician and scientist, I loved finding proof in the numbers that certain beans can deliver greater benefits.

We went on to test roast temperatures and techniques, and found that we could preserve phenols that often are destroyed during the process of roasting green coffee. We came to call the lighter roasts "lean roasts," because they're lean on roast flavor, deliver the most phenols, and are naturally delicious enough to forgo fattening additives. We tested grind sizes and brew techniques to determine how to get the highest extraction of phenols and the best flavor. The lab results that we poured into this book can be found nowhere else. They tell us definitively which coffee beans and preparations produce the best-tasting and healthiest coffees in the world.

In addition to lab testing, I researched countless scientific studies on coffee's role in mood improvement, disease prevention, sports performance, and weight loss. Before long, I was eager to conduct my own study. After testing coffees in the analytical chemistry laboratory for maximum benefits, I wanted to test how they performed in real life. Would they really make people feel better?

I partnered with Dr. David Nieman, director of the Human Performance Lab at the North Carolina Research Campus and professor at Appalachian State University, to conduct a clinical trial that would test the influences of high-phenol coffee on mood and performance. The results (found in chapter 1) of our double-blind, randomized, crossover study amazed us all. Just thirty minutes after drinking high-phenol coffee prepared by the Greek method, participants felt more active, lively, and energetic. Exercise felt much easier. But most profound was this finding: After participants drank a cup of high-phenol coffee each day for two weeks, testing revealed significant improvements in their overall moods, even when measured after overnight fasts, before they drank coffee. High-phenol coffee proved to have the chronic effect of helping people feel more energized and optimistic, without the influence of caffeine.

My most important task had become clear: to convince you to always drink high-phenol coffees made from the very best beans and the leanest roasts. These buoy your mood, fight off illness, and boost your metabolism and cardiovascular function, while spurring weight loss.

Once you know how to select quality beans, we'll teach you several brewing techniques, including the Greek method. The Coffee Lover's Diet will give you a plan for using cof-

BOB ARNOT, M.D.

fee as a ritual, reward, and unparalleled fuel throughout your day. Meals include nutrition-packed chia/fruit smoothies and lean but satisfying foods. You'll find suggestions for pairing coffees with carefully chosen foods, as well as a host of delicious recipes. In addition, you'll learn the most common coffee mistakes (like loading burnt coffee with fat and sugar) and how to avoid coffee's few perils, such as high acrylamide levels and jagged caffeine side effects. We'll bust the myths that have pervaded the coffee story with hard analytical chemistry.

Before you dive in, know your caffeine limit. Nearly half of the human population is genetically slow to metabolize caffeine. You can determine whether you're a fast or slow caffeine metabolizer by ordering a genetic test from companies such as 23andMe.com, but you probably already know which one you are. If more than two cups of caffeinated coffee gives you road rage, makes your heart race, or disturbs your sleep, you're a slow metabolizer. If you can drink espresso after dinner and sleep like a baby, you're probably a fast caffeine metabolizer. To reap any health benefits from poor-quality coffee, you'd have to drink a great deal of it, which is unthinkable and even dangerous to slow metabolizers, like me. We can benefit, however, by drinking high-phenol decaffeinated coffees, or a few cups of well-spaced high-phenol caffeinated coffee, which blunts that jittery feel.

I have totally fallen in love with the world's best coffees, and I've never felt or performed better. If you love coffee, you can delight in knowing that one of your greatest pleasures can also be the healthiest thing you do for yourself each day. If you thought you couldn't enjoy coffee, this book will teach you to safely reap its benefits, from helping you shed extra weight to improving your athletic performance, and even fend off disease.

BOB ARNOT, M.D.

PART I

COFFEE: THE ULTIMATE HEALTH FOOD

CHAPTER 1

THE BENEFITS

THE BENEFITS

From decades of medical research conducted all around the globe, an ancient beverage has emerged as the ultimate health food. The most popular drink in the world after water, coffee can improve mental health, enhance athletic performance, aid weight loss, and offer us resistance to the most ravaging diseases of our time: heart disease, diabetes, cancer, and neurological disorders like Parkinson's disease and Alzheimer's. A vast wealth of new research tells us that the beloved daily ritual of enjoying hot, fragrant, delicious coffee can do more good for us than we ever thought.

Assuming it was bad for me, I stayed away from coffee until about four years ago, when I read in *The New England*

Journal of Medicine about its spectacular health benefits. I began drinking Keurig K-cups; then I progressed to grinding and brewing my own coffee at home. Now coffee has become the greatest nutritional treat in my life. I can hardly go to sleep at night imagining the flavors and aromas I'll experience when dawn breaks and I prepare a new coffee. There's no guilt, because along with all the sensory pleasure, I'm giving myself tremendous health benefits. As you read in the introduction, so powerful are coffee's benefits that *The New England Journal of Medicine* reports that drinking several cups a day reduces the risk of death from all causes by 15 percent in women and by 10 percent in men.[1]

For decades, coffee was associated with poorer health because many coffee drinkers had higher-than-average weights and higher red meat and alcohol consumption, and they smoked and didn't exercise. But this enormous landmark study set aside those risk factors to examine the true effects of coffee, which are far more impressive than any of us had believed.

What's in coffee that gives it a protective effect? Caffeine gets due credit for helping us wake up, but it also raises metabolism, boosts our physical speed and power, and can even make us happier. The true magic in coffee, however, lies in its polyphenols, which make coffee by far the greatest source of antioxidants in the average American diet. (See the chart on page 20.) Some coffee plants produce far more polyphenols than others, making themselves stronger, their beans taste better, and you healthier

BOB ARNOT, M.D.

when you drink them. A perfect trifecta. Coffee is an ideal delivery mechanism for phenols, allowing them to be absorbed easily in the bloodstream, where they can reduce inflammation and oxidation, lower blood sugar, and reduce blood pressure.

These capabilities are profound. As I researched this book, every week, it seemed, new connections were discovered between coffee, fitness, and disease resistance, and the headlines began to follow. Even the World Health Organization has weighed in. Twenty-five years after classifying coffee as a possible carcinogen leading to bladder cancer,[2] the WHO issued a press release announcing the findings of a group of scientists convened by its cancer agency. On June 15, 2016, the international group of twenty-three scientists wrote this in a press release:

> After thoroughly reviewing more than 1,000 studies in humans and animals, the Working Group found that there was inadequate evidence for the carcinogenicity of coffee drinking overall.
>
> Many epidemiological studies showed that coffee drinking had no carcinogenic effects for cancers of the pancreas, female breast, and prostate, and reduced risks were seen for cancers of the liver and uterine endometrium.

With the capabilities of average coffee making such news, imagine the greater potential of coffees with exponentially

TOP TEN SOURCES OF ANTIOXIDANTS IN U.S. DIET

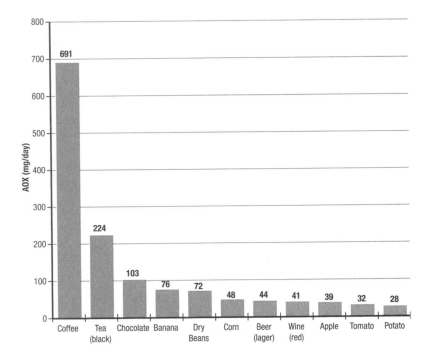

Joe Vinson, Ph.D., at the University of Scranton, published these values for antioxidants consumed in the American diet. Coffee is the clear leader. "Nothing else comes close," says Dr. Vinson.

BOB ARNOT, M.D.

more phenols! This book will teach you how to find these better beans and, just as important, to prepare them in a way that preserves their essential goodness. But, first, let's look at all that coffee can do for you.

COFFEE'S MVP: CGA

Chlorogenic acid, a natural chemical compound found in many plants and foods, may be the polyphenol most beneficial to human health. Naturally present in coffee (although in varying levels), CGAs perform a multitude of helpful actions, but chief among them are reducing inflammation and blocking the jittery effects of caffeine.[3] These actions work hand in hand; CGAs diminish feelings of shakiness, racing hearts, or anxiousness that many people feel after consuming caffeine, allowing those who once felt they couldn't tolerate coffee to reap its anti-inflammatory and antioxidant benefits.

After switching to high-phenol coffee, Dave Engert, an executive from Paradise Valley, Arizona, wrote to me that he gets "a much smoother effect than I usually get from other coffees. In other words, a nice easy acceleration in waking up and getting 'crisp' without a big jolt or the 'jitters.'" CGAs make coffee drinking more tolerable to those who are caffeine sensitive, so they can benefit further from this and other healthy phenols.

There can be no overstating the value of CGA's ability to reduce inflammation, particularly in the United States and other Western cultures, where a preference for refined grains and sugars has driven it to threatening levels. Inflammation makes people feel wretched. Let me paint you a picture of it. You have a wound on your arm that becomes red, swollen, and sore. Soon the infection overwhelms the anti-inflammatory forces in your body, causing a condition that only powerful antibiotics can counter. Imagine this same inflammation living inside your heart, lungs, blood vessels, digestive system, and even your brain. You may not have the same pain you get from an infection on your arm, but you will have symptoms and, eventually, disease. Dysphoria. Depression. Inflammation of the heart's arteries, which can lead to coronary artery disease. Other degenerative illnesses driven by inflammation are

- Cancer
- Diabetes
- Osteoarthritis
- Autoimmune diseases
- Neurodegenerative diseases such as Parkinson's and Alzheimer's

While inflammation doesn't directly cause these diseases, it does trip the master switches that accelerate their onset. CGA wins coffee's most valuable player award because it is so effective at dousing the fires of inflammation. CGA's powerful anti-inflammatory effect makes it a critical combatant of all those diseases with an inflammatory basis, from heart disease to depression. The more CGAs you drink, the more you damp down inflammation.

This is how it happens: Within the body, signaling molecules called eicosanoids regulate inflammation and immune functions. There are good ones and bad ones. The bad ones, called pro-inflammatory eicosanoids, reach sky-high levels when arthritis, infection, and diabetes are present.[4] These eicosanoids trigger redness, swelling, pain, and heat. By contrast, anti-inflammatory eicosanoids diminish inflammation and pain. CGAs help calm inflammation by increasing levels of the anti-inflammatory eicosanoids. You'll find a list of coffees with high levels of CGAs in the Resources section of this book. You can get still more anti-inflammatory eicosanoids by eating certain healthy foods. Omega-3 fish oils, for instance, trigger the formation of anti-inflammatory eicosanoids, while white flours and fried foods generate the inflammatory kind. Eicosanoids and CRP (C-reactive protein) are markers of inflammation that can be easily measured in the blood, so you can find out what your inflammation level is by asking your doctor for a CRP test.

BE HAPPIER

We all know that coffee improves alertness, reaction time, and concentration. But can it actually make you happy? It can. On many levels. Obviously, it feels good to wrap your hands around a warm mug and enjoy delicious smells and tastes. But also at work are both of coffee's most active ingredients, caffeine and phenols. I'm sure most of you are familiar with a good caffeine buzz. It makes you feel energized, clear headed, ready to jump into action. That's enough to make most people feel pretty happy, but there's more. A series of groundbreaking studies has revealed coffee to have tremendous prospects for improved mental health, as coffee drinkers showed lower rates of depression and suicide.

In a large study of 50,739 women, the Harvard School of Public Health (HSPH) observed in 2013 that increasing consumption of caffeinated coffee lowered the risk of depression. The effect seemed to be dose dependent. Michel Lucas, a research fellow in nutrition, concluded that there was a 20 percent lower risk of depression among women who drank four or more cups of caffeinated coffee a day, compared to those who drank very little or none. In this study, decaffeinated coffee, tea, soft drinks, and chocolate didn't appear to protect against depression.

In another study at HSPH, men and women who drank several cups of coffee daily had an astounding 50 percent de-

DEPRESSION RISK REDUCTION

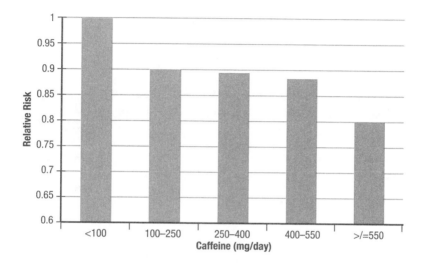

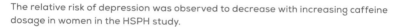

The relative risk of depression was observed to decrease with increasing caffeine dosage in women in the HSPH study.

creased risk of suicide. Published in *The World Journal of Biological Psychiatry,* this study identified caffeine as most likely responsible for the protective effect. Studies in Australia, Finland, and Japan found similar, significant associations between coffee, caffeine, and decreased risk of depression.

Our own study, conducted with North Carolina Research Campus's Dr. David Nieman, one of America's foremost exercise physiologists specializing in human nutrition, found that high-phenol coffee significantly improved participants' overall moods, even when their systems were largely cleared of caffeine.

Our study was a double-blind, placebo-controlled trial, which is the gold-standard design used commonly to prove whether new pharmaceuticals or other therapies work. Double-blind means that neither the subjects nor clinicians knew whether a subject was drinking caffeinated coffee high in CGAs, or a placebo, which was a low-CGA decaf. (Subjects guessed wrong half the time, when asked which they were taking.) We also employed a crossover technique, in which each subject drank one of the two beverages for two weeks, then, following a washout period, drank the other beverage for two weeks. In this way, each subject served as his or her own control. (We chose a two-week period because CGAs may transform bacteria in the large intestine, enabling them to absorb and convert more CGA, so that after two weeks, the body is able to utilize more of this highly anti-inflammatory substance.)

At the end of each two-week trial, we measured participants' TMD, or total mood disturbance, using a standard validated psychological test known as POMS. A series of questions about mood, gauging how tense, anxious, nervous, energetic, or lively subjects feel, POMS stands for Profiles of Mood States. The late Douglas McNair, of the departments of clinical psychopharmacology and psychology at Boston University, developed the test as a means of detecting short-term effects of pharmacologic treatments. The mood instrument was ideal for our study since we were evaluating high-phenol coffee as the equivalent of a therapeutic agent. You can take the test yourself and score it using the POMS questionnaire by BrianMac Sports Coach (https://www .brianmac.co.uk/poms.htm).

WHAT WE FOUND AFTER TWO WEEKS ON HIGH-CGA COFFEE

BEFORE DRINKING HIGH-CGA COFFEE: POMS tests administered in the mornings, after overnight fasts, measured significant improvements in overall mood. The study subjects had consumed no caffeine for twenty-four hours, since the previous morning's coffee, indicating that the chronic effect of the high-CGA coffee was to improve mood even without caffeine. Many of the dieters profiled in this book reported that they experienced improved moods as well, and I've certainly felt it personally. I've never felt more energized or optimistic than I have when drinking these high-phenol coffees daily. Here, finally, is proof of the correlation.

THIRTY MINUTES AFTER DRINKING HIGH-CGA COFFEE: We wanted to find out how quickly high-phenol coffee could improve mood in the short term. Just thirty minutes after subjects drank their coffees, the POMS instrument showed highly significant increases in scores for vigor. The vigor score sums up improvements in indices such as "lively, active, energetic, full of pep, and vigorous." No significant increases of negative feelings, such as "tense, angry, on edge, or uneasy," occurred. Generally, I feel edgy and anxious when I drink low-phenol coffee, but I experience none of these feelings after drinking high-phenol coffee, which is now my go-to morning beverage.

Other study authors, too, have found that, even without caffeine, coffee with high amounts of CGAs can improve mood and cognitive performance.[5] This is great news if you're sensitive to caffeine: A decaf coffee with plenty of CGAs should work as well as caffeinated coffee to help lift your mood. Look for decafs made with Descamex or Swiss Water decaffeination processes, which use water rather than chemicals to remove caffeine. Some decaffeination processes can leach out CGAs, while others leave behind a robust amount, which is why it's important to know the CGA content of your coffee. (In the coming chapters we'll identify which coffees contain the most CGAs.)

HOW IT WORKS

How do phenols work to make you happier? It all comes back to cutting inflammation. You've probably heard of serotonin, the feel-good neurochemical, which first became widely known with the introduction of Prozac.

BOB ARNOT, M.D.

Many antidepressants work by making serotonin more available in the brain. NMDA is another brain chemical, but one associated with depression and chronic pain. Blocking NMDA is a major focus of drug development; in fact, Harvard's famed psychiatry unit at Massachusetts General Hospital runs a depression clinic aimed solely at inhibiting NMDA using a nasal administration of a drug called ketamine. Inflammation diverts a key pathway in the brain so that it manufactures less serotonin and more NMDA. This is really the worst of both worlds, causing inflammation to feed depression. The altered brain chemistry explains why so many Americans with highly inflammatory diets, or inflammatory conditions like obesity and diabetes, feel awful every day.

The good news: Coffee phenols cut inflammation, which helps to restore serotonin production and decrease NMDA production. Many people complain that dieting and exercise make them miserable, but drinking coffee, which is a joy for most of us, can also help us become healthier and happier, by making our brains feel good again.

PERFORM BETTER

Coffee is the ultimate performance-enhancing drug, and it's legal! From getting us up in the morning to fueling our workouts and keeping us on the road at night, it's unparalleled in helping us perform better both mentally and physically.

PHYSICAL PERFORMANCE

Athletes of all levels are catching on to coffee's power to boost performance. Increasingly popular in gyms and among endurance athletes, coffee is a better fuel than sweetened sports beverages, as it has no sugar, few calories, and these incredible capabilities:

- Improves speed and power during exercise
- Preferentially burns fat while you exercise
- Combats oxidation of free radicals

Coffee is the best training aid I've encountered in my years as a competitive Nordic skier, cyclist, marathoner, Ironman participant, alpine racer, and big-ocean stand-up paddler. By increasing your anaerobic threshold, coffee allows you to work at a higher pace, harder and longer than you otherwise might. While you're working harder, longer, and faster, caffeinated coffee can even help you burn fat instead of sugar. Caffeine frees up fatty acids from your fat stores, so you can burn them immediately as fuel. Preserving sugar stores in muscle this way is the secret to going faster and farther in endurance sports.

While helping you burn fat, coffee also can increase speed and power during exercise.

Sports scientists in the United Kingdom studying this potential in coffee discovered groundbreaking results in 2013. As simple a change as drinking coffee an hour before a maximum endurance test, called a time trial, spurred cyclists to ride significantly faster, with notably greater power.[6]

How hard does exercise feel to you? Scientists measure this as perceived exertion. While numerous studies have demonstrated coffee's ability to increase power, speed, and endurance, the research we conducted with Dr. Nieman at NCRC showed that coffee can also make exercise feel easier. We studied high-phenol coffee's influence on performance as well as mood and found amazing results in perceived exertion. An hour after drinking a cup of either high-CGA or placebo coffee, our athletes participated in fifty-kilometer cycling time trials. Thirty minutes into the workouts, when the coffees were exerting their maximum effects, we measured perceived exertion. Athletes who'd had high-CGA coffee found that their workouts felt much easier, even at their highest levels of exertion. The implications of these preliminary findings are simple and powerful: A cup of high-phenol coffee before a workout may make your exercise seem much easier!

We know for certain that coffee can upgrade your athletic performance, but the benefits don't stop there. Coffee also aids recovery. Athletes and exercise fans have known for years that intense and prolonged exercise places a great deal of oxidative and inflammatory stress on the body. The production of energy by muscle cells during exercise generates an excess of one of the most powerful and damaging known oxidants: the superoxide radicals. The harder you exercise and the more oxygen you consume, the more superoxide spews out. This can slow recovery, increase the risk of injury, and decrease the intensity or duration of exercise. With their potent antioxidant properties, the phenols in coffee act as a fire extinguisher to quench superoxides. At the end of our time trials, the cyclists taking high-phenol coffee had higher levels of antioxidants in their blood than those taking the placebo.

Phenols' anti-inflammatory effect supports recovery, too. "They can almost take the place of ibuprofen," says Dr. Nieman. Extensive research has shown that caffeine supports performance by working on the central nervous system, but new studies are focusing on phenols. "The purple color in blueberries, the green in broccoli, all the colors are the polyphenols," explains Dr. Nieman. "Most go to the colon and bacteria break them down. But if you exercise, that opens the door and they come flooding back. They relax the blood vessels to improve blood flow, so the muscle gets better oxygen delivery." You'll read more about how athletes can benefit from coffee in chapter 5, "The Coffee Lover's Diet."

BOB ARNOT, M.D.

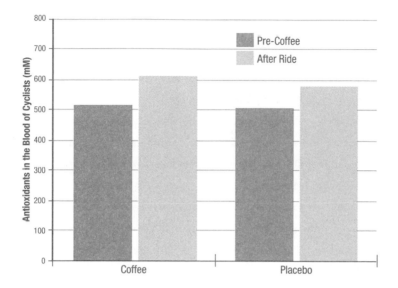

More antioxidants appear in the blood of cyclists who drank high-phenol coffee than a placebo. You see an expected increase in antioxidants after exercise, however, the increase is even greater for high-phenol coffee drinkers than for those drinking the placebo.

DITCH THE JITTERS

Gabriel Beauchesne-Sevigny is on the water by seven thirty almost every morning, digging into Canada's Ottawa River at a rocketing pace. A 2008 Olympian in sprint canoeing, Gabriel doesn't remember a time when he didn't train. "As a kid growing up on the river near my house, I always loved training," he says. "I grew up at the canoe club, and that was my playground." When he was a teenager, Gabriel realized the connection between what he ate and drank, and how he performed.

"I looked for everything that could give me the extra edge and energy," he says. A race may last only four and a half minutes, but training sessions often span two hours. "The quality of my work," he says, "is dependent on my food."

Gabriel liked the energy and alertness that regular coffee gave him in the mornings, but, in trying high-phenol coffee, he found that he could get the results he wanted without the shaky feeling that used to come with them. "I'm ready to go right away," he says. "I'm giving my 100 percent, but the most noticeable thing is: No jitters. No shakes. I have sustained awareness; I'm in the moment, but with no side effects."

This is the work of CGAs, so numerous in high-phenol coffees that they can blunt that jittery feeling, delivering smooth, sustained energy. Gabriel now makes a second cup of high-phenol coffee to drink at three P.M., precisely an hour before his afternoon training, confident in the reliability of the results he'll feel. "When I drink it, I feel great right away, and the effects last a long time."

Tamas Buday, a three-time Olympian in sprint kayaking, also discovered that the smoother energy boost from high-phenol coffee benefits his workouts. A friend and former teammate of Gabriel's, Tamas, too, drinks high-phenol regular coffee before he hits the water. "It picks me up mentally and physically, and I don't get a rush at all," he says. "It really helps pick me up, but relaxes me at the same time. There's a smooth transition later in the day," he adds. "I feel energetic. I might feel fatigued from a workout, but not like I'm crashing from caffeine."

At forty years old, Tamas is on the water daily, working as a full-time canoe and kayak coach for the City of Pointe-Claire in Quebec. After a workout or in the evening, he drinks high-phenol decaf because he enjoys the aroma, flavors, and sense of relaxation it gives him. "It feels good in your system. It's crazy, but it's almost like a recovery drink," he says. Tamas feels just what Dr. Nieman has expressed, that "nature's ibuprofen substitutes are the polyphenols."

STAY HYDRATED

While coffee works wonders as both a fuel and recovery aid, you shouldn't drink only coffee when working out. Water is a must, too. Interestingly, recent reports assert that coffee is not as dehydrating as once was thought; caffeine has a mild diuretic effect, but that is countered by the volume of water in coffee, and also can be negated by exercise.[7] Nonetheless, the common recommendation of eight glasses of water a day remains a good rule of thumb for coffee drinkers. Drink water whenever you're thirsty, and more when you exercise.

MENTAL PERFORMANCE

Now let's see how coffee can crank up your mental game. Uniquely able to increase alertness, coffee has an effect almost like that of a nearsighted person putting on glasses: Suddenly a vague swath of green against the sky becomes a stand of trees bearing thousands of individual leaves.

Help with waking up is the number one reason most of us drink coffee. When we wake, our mental alertness is impaired. We can't focus, we feel as if underwater, we pour orange juice in the cereal. Caffeine overcomes this sleep inertia, clearing the mental fog to make us functional again. By improving attention over a sustained period, and short-

BOB ARNOT, M.D.

ening reaction time, caffeine also helps people stay awake. A 2013 Australian study[8] of long-distance drivers of commercial vehicles showed a 63 percent reduced likelihood of crashing among drivers who drank caffeinated substances, compared with those who did not. Caffeine helps us better focus on the right stimulus, such as an oncoming car, or a child darting into the road. In fact, in keeping drivers alert, two hundred milligrams of caffeine is about as effective as a thirty-minute nap.[9]

Even seventy-five milligrams of caffeine is enough to increase attention over a sustained period of time. You can get that amount in a single cup of coffee, although the FDA cautions that you may get anywhere from sixty to one hundred fifty milligrams in a five-ounce cup. (I like high-altitude Kenyan and Ethiopian coffees because they contain less caffeine than others.) The highest rates of improved attention are found at two hundred milligrams if you don't usually drink caffeine, and at four hundred milligrams if you drink it every day. You can read more about appropriate levels of caffeine consumption at the end of this chapter.

HOW THE WORLD'S MOST POPULAR PSYCHOACTIVE DRUG WORKS: THE SLEEPY SWITCH

Caffeine acts on the brain primarily by attaching to adenosine receptors so that adenosine cannot. When adenosine attaches, it exerts an inhibitory effect on the central nervous system that leaves us feeling tired or drowsy, which is what I call the sleepy switch. The reason that we feel stimulated after drinking a cup of caffeinated coffee is that caffeine has blocked adenosine from attaching to those receptors, effectively turning off the switch. Caffeine subsequently stimulates production of several neurotransmitters, including dopamine and glutamate. Dopamine is a reward chemical in the brain and the target of many psychopharmacological and recreational drugs. Meanwhile, caffeine also can boost production of adrenaline,[10] making us feel more energized and attentive (but potentially jumpy and anxious if we drink too much too quickly, or metabolize it slowly).

HELP YOUR HEART

Heart disease remains the number one killer in the United States and much of the Western world, so it's no surprise that coffee's ability to reduce risk factors for the disease may be its most widely reported benefit. The landmark study published by *The New England Journal of Medicine* in 2012

BOB ARNOT, M.D.

in 2012 showed that heavy coffee drinkers were 22 percent less likely to die from heart disease than the people who didn't drink coffee. Phenols are the most likely providers of the protection, the authors wrote. The level of protection keeps increasing as coffee intake increases, but few people can drink great quantities of coffee. An extraordinary solution lies in the breakthrough message of this book: You can get exponentially more phenols in a single cup of coffee. The coming chapters will teach you how to maximize the health benefits of coffee without overloading on caffeine. Already you've seen how phenols can reduce inflammation, which can account for up to 50 percent of your risk for heart disease. Let's look now at the influence of coffee phenols on other risk factors, like vascular health, cholesterol, and blood pressure.

VASCULAR HEALTH

To take care of your heart, you must also take care of the vascular system that feeds it. How long do you think it would take to make this system healthier? A year? A month? How about a few hours? Medical testing of the lining of our blood vessels, which is called the endothelium, is emerging as an excellent barometer of vascular health. These tests of endothelial cell function (ECF) have revealed that our blood vessels respond very quickly to what we drink, so they're becoming the new standard for testing the health effects of beverages. In these tests, premium coffees that are flush with antioxidants and anti-inflammatory compounds have proven to make robust, positive changes in vascular health in just a few hours. Of course, getting these benefits requires having sufficient phenols in the coffee you drink. A low-phenol coffee, overroasted and dressed up with fat and sugar, will not serve you well. Some studies have shown consumption of caffeinated coffee to *reduce* endothelial function. Those results may stem from a lack of phenols in the coffee, or from too much caffeine counteracting the positive effect of phenols on ECF.

ECF tests measure how blood vessels react to stress, in order to determine how sick or healthy they are. In a poor reaction, vessels contract, constricting the flow of blood; in a healthy reaction, they expand, letting blood flow to tissues that have been deprived of oxygen. The results of my own ECF test astonished me. After taking a baseline reading, I drank a glass of water with green tea extract, and chased it with my morning smoothie, containing kale, blueberries, cantaloupe, and chia. We waited an hour and retested. I could barely believe my eyes, as my endothelial function boomed. It was nearly 40 percent higher than it was at baseline, before I consumed my beverage!

The study on the longevity of Ikarians that so inspired me found that the islanders who drank Greek coffee had better endothelial function than those who drank other types.

BOB ARNOT, M.D.

The more Greek coffee the islanders drank, the better their endothelial function became. This was the first solid indication that coffee can improve ECF. Brimming with phenols, the Greek coffee produced a positive effect on ECF even in patients who had high blood pressure, high cholesterol, diabetes, or smoked.

"Boiled Greek type of coffee, which is rich in polyphenols and antioxidants and contains only a moderate amount of caffeine, seems to gather benefits compared to other coffee beverages," wrote one of the study authors, Dr. Gerasimos Siasos.

Impressed with my ECF results and once again inspired by the Ikarians, I began testing volunteers. One was a young man in his midthirties who had no obvious signs of poor health, but an extraordinary risk of heart disease. His reactive hyperemia index (RHI), a measurement of blood flow after temporary blockage, was 159, on the borderline of a poor result. He drank a cup of a lightly roasted, finely ground Kenyan Karogoto coffee. An hour later, his RHI was 220, and he felt dramatically better. Although this research is just beginning, our early findings have been compelling. We gave volunteers a high-fat meal; some drank a high-phenol coffee with it and others did not. Then, using the gold-standard ECF test called flow mediated dilation, as well as RHI, we measured their endothelial function. We found that the high-fat food caused a significant deterioration in ECF; but, in the first several subjects who drank high-phenol coffee with the meal, ECF did not deteriorate, and even improved.

CHEESEBURGER, FRIES, SODA, AND YOUR VASCULAR HEALTH

Foods and beverages can have fast-acting, negative effects on endothelial function, too. Let's imagine that you've just downed a hamburger smothered with cheese and sautéed onions. Add to it French fries and a thirty-two-ounce cola. Now let's watch the action. (Think about this the next time you order a burger.)

FAT: As fat starts to pour into your bloodstream, your endothelial cells are quick to react. Your arteries begin to constrict, limiting the flow of blood.

SUGAR: The vast beds of small vessels that help clear sugar from your blood may begin to close off, allowing your blood sugar to build to dangerous levels.

BLOOD CLOTS: Your meal makes platelets stickier, so they are more likely to clump together. Clumps of platelets are the beginnings of blood clots, and if you have an already damaged artery, a clot could lead to a heart attack. Even after a single bad meal, a diseased coronary artery can begin to contract, and even go into spasm. That's how dynamically your body changes in reaction to unhealthy foods or drinks. It's also why you read stories of people keeling over at the dinner table!

INFLAMMATION: With chronic consumption of highly inflammatory foods like these, you may become dysphoric and even depressed, since inflammation in the brain slows the production of the feel-good neurotransmitter serotonin.

TRIGLYCERIDES: After meals, a fat called triglyceride pours out of your intestine and into your bloodstream. As the triglyceride level climbs in your blood, vessels become less responsive, and ECF falters.

CHOLESTEROL DEPOSITS: As cholesterol from the food is deposited inside artery walls, they become stiff and in-flexible over time.

Foods and drinks like these punish our bodies, depriving our blood vessels of the ability to respond to stress, and making us sick. If we eat them often, inflammation and harmful oxidants make our mood plummet, and destroy the chemical synthesis that occurs in the endothelium. People tend to think of nutrition as having a cumulative ef-fect over time, but, as the work with ECF and coffee shows, significant changes can occur within hours of consuming a meal or beverage.

NITRIC OXIDE

This molecule is a powerful protector of the vascular system. Nitric oxide dilates blood vessels, inhibits platelet aggregation, reduces adhesion of cells to vessel walls, and inhibits growth of new muscle cells within arteries—all of which deter coronary artery disease. In cutting inflammation, which slows the body's production of nitric oxide, CGAs allow nitric oxide to flourish. Phenols in coffee, tea, cocoa, and virgin olive oil enhance production of this beneficial molecule.

CHOLESTEROL

Your doctor has probably discussed LDL (low-density lipoprotein) cholesterol with you. This is what we call bad cholesterol. Bad becomes worse when LDL is oxidized, either in the blood or in the lining of the blood vessels, magnifying its effects and accelerating the onset of atherosclerosis. One likely reason that studies show a lower risk of coronary artery disease in coffee drinkers[11] is that CGAs inhibit the oxidation of LDL in the blood and below the surface of blood vessels, where cholesterol deposits form. CGAs also decrease concentrations of cholesterol and triglycerides in blood and tissue. Generally, they provide an overall boost to the antioxidant capability of the blood as it courses through the body.

While coffee can lower cholesterol in this way, unfiltered

coffees may actually increase it, as some Scandinavian studies have shown. Unfiltered coffees allow fats that are typically trapped by filters to pass into the cup. These fats, one of which, you may remember, is called cafestol, offer excellent anti-inflammatory value, but consuming too many of them can raise cholesterol. It seems a tricky choice that faces fans of unfiltered coffee, but a simple solution is to enjoy just one or two cups of unfiltered high-phenol coffee a day, switch to filtered if you want additional coffees, and keep close track of cholesterol.

STOP OXIDATION

Inflammation's mean sidekick, oxidation, is another major driving force of illness in the body. To visualize oxidation, think of an old car bumper. The ugly rash of rust on the bumper is the work of strong oxidation. If oxidation can devour a car, think of what it can do to the inside of your body. It wreaks havoc by hacking away at your DNA. The phenols in coffee, the most prevalent antioxidants in the American diet, provide an excellent buffer against oxidation, which, in turn, is good for the heart.

BLOOD PRESSURE

High blood pressure is perhaps one of the best-known symptoms of potential heart trouble. CGA, seemingly limitless in its power to do good in your body, evidently can lower blood pressure as well. Animal studies came first; in 2006 scientists determined that the more CGAs animals consumed, the lower their blood pressure became. Then they replicated these results in humans. After twenty-eight days of drinking green coffee extract, which is extremely high in CGAs, the people in the study experienced decreases in blood pressure.[12]

Caffeine and hydroxyhydroquinone (HHQ), another substance in coffee produced during roasting, can counter this antihypertensive effect of CGA, so don't overdo the caffeine. To reduce HHQ, use a charcoal filter and choose lighter roasts. For those of us who are slow to metabolize caffeine, caffeinated coffee may even raise blood pressure, so choosing superior decafs is vital to deriving the benefits of coffee.

NEVER TOO LATE

Even after a heart attack, habitual coffee drinking can reduce the risk of death. A recent study in the UK, published in *Coronary Artery Disease*, observed a significant inverse correlation between coffee drinking and mortality following heart attacks. Light coffee drinkers had 79 percent of the chance of death that non-coffee drinkers had, and heavy coffee drinkers had a stunning 54 percent of the chance of death of nondrinkers.

LOSE THE WEIGHT

If you're reading this book, you probably love coffee, or want to get rid of some extra weight, or both. Given the overwhelming interest in (and need for) weight loss in our country, it stuns me that for so long we overlooked coffee's ideal role as a diet aid. Chapter 5, "The Coffee Lover's Diet," will deliver much more information on how to use coffee to help you lose weight, but here we'll give you a preview of this most sought-after benefit.

No other food or beverage can do as much as coffee to activate weight loss. Coffee does all this, and more:

- Tastes great
- Contains two calories per cup
- Burns fat

- Raises metabolism
- Provides extra energy
- Improves blood sugar
- Decreases fat absorption
- Prevents weaponization of fat

Good coffees can taste like nuts, chocolate, berries, honey, and a host of other wonderful things. Because they're delicious without cream or sugar, they are nearly calorie-free rewards you can enjoy throughout the day, so you have something to look forward to, as well as something to distract you from destructive snacking. Meanwhile, as you've seen, coffee can put you in a better mood—something we all need when dieting!

While coffee helps you beat the mental challenges of dieting, it is unparalleled at triggering weight loss physically. Caffeine increases the body's metabolic rate,[13] so you burn more calories even when you're not exercising. When you do exercise, coffee can wrest better results from each workout. Remember, drinking coffee an hour before you work out not only gives you more energy, speed, and power, it helps you selectively burn fat as a fuel. This fat-burning capability, which frees fatty acids from your fat stores to burn in place of sugar, is a phenomenal boost to weight loss.

Coffee's a fat buster in still other ways. Phenols help reduce the body's production of new fat, while melanoidin, a valuable antioxidant in coffee, works in the digestive system to decrease

BOB ARNOT, M.D.

the absorption of some fats. I suspect this is the reason people instinctively reach for coffee after big, fatty dinners. While in the gut, these melanoidins also prevent fat peroxidation—what I call the weaponization of fat—a process that creates more dangerous fats that can damage cell membranes and contribute to the risk of coronary artery disease.

SUCCESS!

A fellow resident of my idyllic winter hometown of Stowe, Vermont, Chris Goss already lived a pretty healthy lifestyle, dining on big, fresh salads and lean proteins with his wife, an energetic amateur athlete. Nevertheless, Chris, like so many people, felt locked in a pattern of losing and regaining the same twenty pounds. For the fifty-two-year-old director of hospitality at Stowe Mountain Resort, sometimes a lack of time for exercise was to blame, sometimes work-related stress, sometimes just an indulgence in flaky baguettes alongside meals.

Coffee is a longtime love for Chris, so, having read the research on its intrinsic benefits to wellness and weight loss, he was eager to try the Coffee Lover's Diet.

"It takes three to five minutes at the most to make the smoothies," Chris says. He would make a large smoothie and take it to business meetings in the mornings along with his insulated cup of coffee. "It was easier to eat lean because I had the smoothie to keep my stomach full. And eating lean was easier knowing I got to sip on this great coffee throughout the day, and I didn't have to limit myself," he adds. Meanwhile, Chris was exercising four to five days a week, doing forty minutes of aerobic exercise along with stretching and strengthening work.

In sixty days, Chris had lost eighteen pounds. Bonus results, he says, were increased energy, suppressed appetite, and positive mood benefits. The best result of all, however, may have come when, as he puts it, he "fell off the program." A stressful time brought Chris's exercise and smoothies to a halt. He didn't drastically change his meal content, though, and he continued drinking several cups of high-phenol coffee a day.

Chris went to his doctor for a physical. He was regretting having fallen off the program. But, he says, "I was totally surprised when I got on the scale." He'd regained only five pounds. The features that make coffee the ideal dieter's food, from increasing metabolism to burning more fat during exercise, even walking, may have helped Chris avoid regaining more weight. "In the past I would've ballooned back up. I would've felt bloated and puffy," he says. This time, with only five pounds to lose, Chris felt confident that he could easily get back to where he wanted to be.

BOB ARNOT, M.D.

DEFY DIABETES

Poor dietary choices and a lack of exercise can lead to the development of type 2 diabetes. Of the nearly twenty-six million Americans who have diabetes, 90 to 95 percent have type 2, which is largely *preventable* with healthy lifestyle habits.[14] Controlling weight and blood sugar are crucial to fending off this disease, which can cause debilitating, potentially lethal conditions from head to foot. Here, too, coffee, is a heavy hitter, helping to defy diabetes by lowering blood sugar, improving insulin response after meals, and cutting down inflammation. Thanks to these effects, coffee drinkers have lower incidence of type 2 diabetes than non–coffee drinkers, according to numerous studies.

DRINK HIGH-PHENOL COFFEE TO LOWER YOUR BLOOD SUGAR IN THREE WAYS

1. Increase insulin sensitivity: CGAs help the insulin in your body work better, so you require less of it.[15, 16, 17]
2. Clear blood sugar: CGAs decrease absorption of sugar in the intestine.
3. Slow sugar production: CGAs slow production of sugar in the liver.

One impressive study, conducted recently[18] in Athens, Greece, followed more than three thousand men and women over ten years, and found that those who consumed more than 250 milliliters, or roughly a cup, of coffee a day had 54 percent lower odds of developing diabetes. Little more than a cup of coffee each day *cut in half* their odds of getting this disease!

Yet another study, conducted by Chinese scientists in 2014, found that coffee could reduce the incidence of adult-onset diabetes.[19] This study showed that the chance of diabetes decreased by 12 percent for every two cups of regular coffee subjects added to their daily intake. For decaf, there was an 11 percent decrease in risk for every two cups added per day. The effects are even better among those who are lean and don't smoke.

Several of the diabetes studies credit coffee's anti-inflammatory traits for its protective effect. A classic study published in *The American Journal of Clinical Nutrition*[20] tested the blood of 730 healthy women and 663 with type 2 diabetes. The study showed that in women with diabetes, coffee drinking decreased their markers for inflammation, such as CRP. Just as important, these women had less dysfunction of the endothelium. In the healthy women, decaf coffee decreased inflammation as well as regular, which indicated the anti-inflammatory benefits of phenols.

CGA isn't the only compound in coffee that helps deter diabetes. Cafestol, a type of fat known as a diterpene that we discussed earlier, is a healthy fat that can increase insulin sensitivity and improve glucose clearance, making it highly useful in the treatment and prevention of diabetes. Again, cafestol can raise your cholesterol if you consume too much of it, but since it can be beneficial in moderate amounts, try the unfiltered coffee preparations, which allow cafestol to pass into the coffee. (You'll learn these techniques in chapter 4.) Do check first with your doctor if you have high cholesterol.

REDUCE YOUR RISK OF CANCER

As public opinion swings from one extreme to another, isn't it nice when you find that science is pushing the pendulum? The medical community has examined carefully any possible links between cancer and coffee. In fact, the American Institute for Cancer Research puts the number of studies on the topic at more than one thousand. "Early in the research, some studies hinted that coffee might increase cancer risk. Larger and more well-designed studies now suggest the opposite: it may be protective for some cancers," the institute reports.[21] Sea changes like these don't take hold without evidence; some of the more recent studies followed tens of thousands of subjects over more than a decade. They've found that, in many cases, the more cups of coffee consumed per day, the greater the reduction of risk.

Scientific Reports,[22] a part of the prestigious Nature Publishing Group, recently published an analysis of 105 prospective studies. The review concluded that there is a reduced risk of oral, pharynx, liver, colon, prostate, and endometrial cancers among coffee drinkers. While the *Scientific Reports* analysis indicated that there may be an increased risk of lung cancer for coffee drinkers, a separate analysis of lung cancer studies showed no increased risk for coffee drinkers who are nonsmokers.[23]

NEUROPROTECTION

Alzheimer's is a disease that terrifies most of us as we age. While excellent treatments exist for heart disease and many cancers, we can do little to stem the onset of Alzheimer's disease, which is the most common cause of dementia. Its prevalence is staggering. In the United States, one in every nine people over the age of sixty-five suffers from Alzheimer's.[24] For the year 2016, the Alzheimer's Association estimated the cost of treating this disease and other dementias to be $236 billion. There is good news, however: Drinking coffee over the course of your lifetime lowers your risk of developing this terrible disease.

This notion brought me back to the people of Ikaria, the vast majority of whom stay mentally sharp to the ends of their long lives. The Ikarians have only about *a quarter* of our rate of dementia in the United States. Surely their diets, lifestyles, and social networks contribute to this enviable clarity of mind, but, given the spate of studies linking ordinary coffee to reduced risk of Alzheimer's, I suspect their phenol-packed Greek coffee helps, too.

HOW DOES IT WORK?

The theory goes like this: In early stages of Alzheimer's, clusters of beta-amyloid molecules bind strongly to receptors on nerve cells, sparking a process that erodes their synapses with other nerve cells.[25] Caffeine blocks those receptors so that the beta-amyloid can't attach to them.

The Institute for Scientific Information on Coffee, a resource site for health care providers in England, has surveyed many studies on coffee and Alzheimer's, which found clearly reduced risks of Alzheimer's for coffee drinkers. A 2015 Italian study found among older individuals who habitually drank moderate amounts of coffee (one to two cups a day) a lower incidence of mild cognitive impairment than in those who never or rarely drank coffee.[26]

Scientists also have observed a substantially reduced risk of Parkinson's disease among coffee drinkers. Another neurodegenerative disorder, Parkinson's strikes sixty thousand Americans each year. It produces tremors, drags down motor function, and destroys neurons in the brain. Happily, researchers found, when analyzing a group of twenty different studies, that the global risk of developing Parkinson's disease decreased by 31 percent in coffee drinkers compared to non–coffee drinkers. In analyzing another group of twenty-six studies on the topic, the risk of coffee drinkers developing Parkinson's was 25 percent lower than the risk for non–coffee drinkers.[27]

Coffee drinking may also protect against strokes. After following thousands of women for an average of ten years, a study run by Susanna Larsson of the Karolinska Institutet in Stockholm found that women who drank more than one cup of coffee a day had 22 percent to 25 percent lower risk of stroke than those who drank less. The association is even stronger in those who don't smoke. The comprehensive study even indicated that those who drank little or no coffee had a slightly increased risk of stroke.[28]

NEUROPROTECTION IN ACTION

Maintaining a healthy cardiovascular system is especially important to Beth M., a political consultant in Boston. Two years ago, Beth, who is in her fifties, suffered a brain hemorrhage. Fully recovered but concerned about the possibility of another bleed, she does everything she can to keep her blood pressure low and strengthen her cardiovascular system.

After her recovery, Beth began drinking high-phenol

coffee for its protective benefits. "I put great importance on an anti-inflammatory and antioxidant diet, and it's fabulous to start my day with a kick of antioxidants in my absolutely delicious cup of [high-phenol] coffee," she says.

Having never had a glass of Coke in her life, and rarely a caffeinated beverage of any kind, Beth drinks strictly high-phenol decaf. She takes with her on vacation her premium beans and minigrinder. Overall, the targeted changes in her diet have Beth feeling great. "My antioxidant, anti-inflammatory dietary regimen keeps my energy up, reduces aches and pains, and has led me to feel stronger than I have in years. It's hard to attribute all of this just to the coffee alone, but I definitely feel my coffee is an important part of the program," she says.

WHO CAN BENEFIT FROM COFFEE?

PARTIERS: If you party hard, you're punishing your brain and liver. The antioxidant, anti-inflammatory actions of coffee can help save you from yourself by protecting both. Coffee won't get you safely home, though, so call an Uber!

BIG EATERS: Say you just devoured a huge steak and a mountain of French fries. You certainly enjoyed yourself, but you're going to pay a price. A medium-roast, high-phenol coffee can help blunt the damage, by decreasing the amount of fat you absorb, by making the fat that sneaks into your system less lethal, by helping to clear your blood sugar, and by safeguarding your vascular function.

ATHLETES: No one benefits from coffee more than athletes, for whom it delivers higher power, speed, and endurance.

ENERGY DRINK ENTHUSIASTS: Coffee loaded with phenols delivers smooth energy and mobilizes extra fuel from your fat stores for daylong energy.

THOSE AT RISK FOR CANCER: Many studies have observed that coffee drinking is associated with a reduced risk of cancers across the spectrum. Coffee won't eradicate the origin of cancers, but it may dampen the inflammation that might drive cancer growth and the oxidation that damages your DNA. Nevertheless, don't forgo regular screenings.

DIABETICS: Along with good nutrition and a healthy lifestyle, coffee can help prevent the onset of type 2 diabetes. Analysis of a host of studies concluded that every additional cup of coffee consumed in a day was associated with a 7 percent reduction in the risk of diabetes.[29]

THOSE AT RISK FOR HEART DISEASE: Coffee drinkers have a lower risk of heart disease than nondrinkers, reports *The New England Journal of Medicine* and numerous other publications. Polyphenols in coffee improve several factors that threaten the heart, from cholesterol and blood pressure to the stickiness of platelets that can stop up arteries.

THE SHORT OF SLEEP: Coffee improves alertness, concentration, memory, and performance on cognitive tasks, making driving safer and improving performance at work or school.[30] (However, as a new Department of Defense blog warns, consuming excessive caffeine can hurt the quality of your sleep and leave you tired. They suggest limiting caffeine to two hundred milligrams in a four-hour period.)

THOSE IN NEED OF A MOOD LIFT: Coffee can pick up your mood immediately and improve it long-term. (If you're depressed, get first-rate professional help.)

CAFFEINE SAVVY

We've now seen some impressive study findings that link coffee to life-changing improvements in health, fitness, and weight loss. In some of them, subjects drank several cups of coffee a day, however, which could be dangerous for some of us. Caffeine is the most widely used psychoactive drug in the world; the American Society for Nutrition reports that 89 percent of adults in the United States consume it on a daily basis. But roughly half of the human population is genetically slow to metabolize caffeine, which renders its effects more pronounced and longer lasting. There are a few variants of an allele on a gene known as *CYP1A2*, which encodes for a liver enzyme that metabolizes caffeine. The allele you carry determines your tolerance of caffeine. Typically, caffeine has a half-life between five and six hours, which is the length of time it takes to metabolize half of the caffeine in your system. If you're a slow caffeine metabolizer, however, this may take your body ten or more hours.

In conducting our research at NCRE, we found that traces of caffeine can remain present in the blood for more than twenty-four hours. We gave fifteen coffee drinkers a single cup of coffee containing 400 milligrams of caffeine, which is the upper limit of daily consumption suggested by the FDA. The participants were restricted from drinking any more caffeine for twenty-four hours, after which we took blood samples. To my surprise, every one of them still had caffeine in his or her system. The fast metabolizers had as little as 1,674 nanograms per milliliter. However, the slow metabolizers had more than 17,000 nanograms per milliliter—as much as if they had just drunk a normal cup of coffee. This finding may explain why so many Americans sleep poorly; their blood is loaded with caffeine all night long!

The famed *New England Journal of Medicine* study found that the more coffee the participants drank, the more they

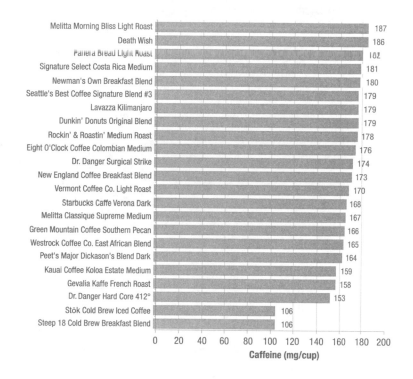

Coffee	Caffeine (mg/cup)
Melitta Morning Bliss Light Roast	187
Death Wish	186
Panera Bread Light Roast	182
Signature Select Costa Rica Medium	181
Newman's Own Breakfast Blend	180
Seattle's Best Coffee Signature Blend #3	179
Lavazza Kilimanjaro	179
Dunkin' Donuts Original Blend	179
Rockin' & Roastin' Medium Roast	178
Eight O'Clock Coffee Colombian Medium	176
Dr. Danger Surgical Strike	174
New England Coffee Breakfast Blend	173
Vermont Coffee Co. Light Roast	170
Starbucks Caffe Verona Dark	168
Melitta Classique Supreme Medium	167
Green Mountain Coffee Southern Pecan	166
Westrock Coffee Co. East African Blend	165
Peet's Major Dickason's Blend Dark	164
Kauai Coffee Koloa Estate Medium	159
Gevalia Kaffe French Roast	158
Dr. Danger Hard Core 412°	153
Stōk Cold Brew Iced Coffee	106
Steep 18 Cold Brew Breakfast Blend	106

Caffeine (mg/cup)

The Coffee Lab (you can find more information on coffeechemlab.com) tested a range of popular coffees from grocery stores and Amazon sales for caffeine content. Death Wish was near the top of the list, verifying their claim as one of the world's strongest coffees. Dr. Danger Hard Core ranked the lowest among roast coffees, which is typical of Ethiopian coffees.

lowered their risk of all causes of death. A recent study on slow caffeine metabolizers, however, showed that, for them, increasing caffeine intake could increase the risk of nonfatal heart attack.[31] To safely reap the many benefits of coffee, we recommend drinking the high-phenol coffees you'll read about in the next chapter. You can get more phenols in one cup of these coffees than in ten cups of a low-phenol coffee. I'm a slow caffeine metabolizer, so I usually drink a half cup of high-phenol regular coffee in the morning, and no more than one or two cups, then switch to high-phenol decaf.

How much caffeine should you consume? According to the FDA, four hundred milligrams a day—that's about four or five cups of coffee—is an amount "not generally associated with dangerous, negative effects." (More than six hundred milligrams per day is too much, they say; average consumption in the United States is about three hundred milligrams a day.) If you feel anxious, can't sleep at night, or find your heart rate racing, you're likely getting too much caffeine. At a recent meeting, a Harvard neurologist told me that the first thing she tells anxious patients is to decrease their coffee consumption. Be aware, though, that coffee isn't your only source of caffeine; you may consume it in jelly beans, gum, water, syrup, and even waffles.[32] A cup of decaf has only two to five milligrams of caffeine, but that is enough to disturb sleep if drunk in the evening. Remember that caffeine reaches its maximum blood level about an hour after consumption and the effects typically last between four and six hours.

The first step in monitoring your caffeine intake is to

know how much of it is in your coffee. The table on page 61 gives you a peek at the caffeine content of several coffees we tested in the lab, but you can find the caffeine content of most coffees through a quick online search.

Thanks to decades of scientific study across numerous fields, we now know that drinking moderate amounts of coffee can bring us a host of meaningful benefits. Coffee can make us happier. It can help us lose weight, maximize our exercise, lower our risk of whole categories of illnesses. All coffees are not created equally, however, so in moving on, we'll identify which beans can deliver the highest return on these incredible benefits. We'll explore the nuances of coffee roasting, and learn to prevent destruction of the antioxidant and anti-inflammatory compounds that are inherent in good coffee. We'll teach you to make yourself the biggest-benefit, best-tasting coffee you've ever had, and identify amazing foods with which to pair it.

PART II

CHANGE YOUR COFFEE, CHANGE YOUR LIFE

THE DIRTY DOZEN: TOP TWELVE COFFEE MISTAKES

1. ADDING SUGAR

Buy and brew better coffee, and skip the sugar! Your blood, your brain, and your belly will thank you.

2. ADDING CREAM

Don't buy roasts so dark they need milk products to be drinkable. A lighter roast will deliver natural flavors that you won't want to mask with milk. And I bet you'll notice a difference when you step on the scale!

3. BUYING VERY DARK-ROASTED COFFEE

Very dark roasts destroy coffee's most beneficial components and lead most people to pad their diets and waistlines with cream and sugar.

4. BUYING BAD COFFEE

Premium coffee from farms with good cultivation practices that are located at high altitudes, near the equator, will taste great and make you feel better. Subscribe to coffeereview.com for help in finding them, and see our list of recommended beans in the Resources section of this book.

5. USING DIRTY EQUIPMENT

Your coffee will taste better if you wash your equipment regularly. Run a cleansing brew now and then with hot water and white vinegar.

6. USING PREGROUND BEANS

There is no way to make a fresh cup of coffee when you buy preground beans. Buy whole beans and grind them just before brewing for the freshest-tasting coffee.

7. USING OLD BEANS

Buy only what you need for one to two weeks, so your coffee doesn't go stale.

8. REFRIGERATING COFFEE BEANS

The moisture that can form on refrigerated or frozen beans stales them instantly—and there's a strong chance your beans may taste like your leftover salmon. Store your coffee in an opaque, airtight container in a dark, dry place.

9. GRINDING TO THE WRONG SIZE

Too fine a grind gives you bitter coffee. Too coarse a grind makes it weak, and won't extract your coffee's phenols.

10. USING THE WRONG COFFEE-TO-WATER RATIO

The best cups of coffee start with a specific recipe, not a little-of-this, dash-of-that approach. This mistake is easy to avoid by weighing coffee and water on a scale. Weight is a better measurement than volume.

11. WRONG WATER TEMPERATURE

Water that is too cool makes coffee that is too mellow. Water that is too hot will burn your coffee.

12. WRONG WATER

Cut the chlorine and minerals from your coffee. Use spring or filtered water.

CHAPTER 2

THE BEANS

Long before I had any interest in coffee, I went to East Africa as a young medical student to take an elective at Kenya's Kakamega Provincial General Hospital and a mission clinic in Mumias through the Harvard School of Public Health. During my stay, I set out with a classmate to summit Mt. Kenya, the second-highest peak in Africa after Kilimanjaro. More than seventeen thousand feet high, Mt. Kenya is where British alpine teams trained to climb Mt. Everest in the 1920s and '30s. My friend and I were ambitious young athletes; we arrived from sea level and raced for the top, ignoring warnings from experts to go slowly. Soon we found ourselves with pounding headaches and coughing up a pink froth. Both were sure signs of altitude sickness, which we'd learned in class is a rapidly lethal condition. We quickly reversed course and headed for the valley floor, but there was a catch.

We'd been given a ride past a dangerous game reserve, where locals told us an expatriate had been stomped to death by elephants. We were supposed to be picked up where we'd been dropped off, but were too sick to wait, so on we charged. First, we were treed by a mother elephant and her calves. Then we ran into the most dangerous animal in Africa, a cape buffalo. We followed the advice of our host, the legendary Hilary Hook, a white hunter and former British Army colonel, who had counseled us to take one step forward and then three back to signal that we were not afraid, but would cede to the wild beast. We made it past the cape buffalo and down to the valley, only to hear a tremendous crashing through the bamboo forest. More elephants. We ran at a breakneck pace and returned, finally, to the vast Hook estate. We recovered there, marveling at how the splendid gardens and fine colonial furnishings, amazing food and exquisite local coffee formed an enclave of civility amidst the wild.

That adventure marked the start of a lifelong love of East Africa for me. I didn't know it then, but the coffee plantations we'd crossed through in our mad descent were at an unusually high altitude for coffee, providing plants with a tremendous challenge to survive the elements. Many decades later, it was in that very region, near the foothills of Mt. Kenya, that I learned how vastly better some coffee beans are than others.

It may seem a relatively inconsequential discovery, but it set me on an exciting new path, exploring the link between coffee and better health and fitness. In the following chapters we'll examine the best roasting, grinding, and brewing techniques for making delicious coffee loaded with antioxidants, but all the potential begins with the beans. Selecting the finest beans at the very start of the journey from farm to cup is the most critical step in making coffee work for you, rather than against you.

BETTER BEANS

Picked from the plant and extracted from the cherry, coffee beans are either packed with powerful nutrients or they're not. After that, any number of things can diminish a bean's quality, but at no point can value be added. How different can two beans be? In the analytical chemistry testing that we conducted for this book, we found that a roasted Kenyan bean called SL 28 contained 24,408 milligrams per kilogram of a specific beneficial chlorogenic acid called 3-CQA. By contrast, some coffees we plucked from supermarket shelves held as little as 1,800 milligrams per kilogram of 3-CQA. Coffees like that deliver negligible benefits. This discrepancy among beans is one of the most important, yet least known, facts about coffee today. The brew you drink each morning may offer you nothing but a dose of caffeine, while coffees with high phenol content can bring tremendous benefits, from protection against major illnesses to improved athletic performance. Which one would you rather drink?

Well, it depends how they taste, right? Amazingly, you don't have to choose between big benefits and out-of-this-world taste, as we found a one-to-one correlation between health scores and taste scores in top coffee reviews. This means that the healthiest coffees are also the most delicious!

THE COFFEE HUNTER

Exploration has fascinated me since grade school. Bored to tears while my poor teacher droned on about English grammar, I would sit behind my third-grade desk, covertly consuming geography books and poring over maps of European exploration of Africa. Not since delving into Sir Richard Burton's discovery of the Nile's headwaters have I felt so captivated by a project as I have with hunting the world's best coffees. Coffee beans tell an amazing story that weaves through history and around the globe, as they are rooted in fabled regions like Kenya's Aberdare mountain range and the shores of Lake Kivu in Rwanda, the long-ago source of the Nile. Searching out coffees with the highest levels of phenols gave me the sense of adventure and discovery the early explorers must have felt. I was hunting one of nature's greatest treasures, and I was hooked. I pulled out topographical maps, read through the entire scientific literature on coffee chemistry, and interviewed growers, buyers, scouts, Q-grade cuppers (expert tasters), and scientists around the world.

I met fascinating people who shared their wealth of knowledge about all things coffee. Excited about coffee's potential to improve wellness, they helped me pinpoint its source. Like scientists scouring tropical rain forests for plants with medicinal qualities, we searched for coffees that would prove in the lab to reduce inflammation and prevent disease. Where would they be? We tried to think like a coffee plant. Where does it most need to defend itself? At high altitudes, close to the equator, a coffee plant faces the harshest ultraviolet rays and lowest temperatures. Here, the plant has to form the strongest defenses. Challenged to be its very best by cold nights and harsh sun, the bean, or seed, grows more robust by producing phenols. High altitudes also cause coffee beans to mature more slowly and become denser than those grown closer to sea level. This slow maturation produces very rich flavor. Ultimately, the seeds that are driven to protect themselves with the strongest antioxidant defenses mature slowly into dense, hard beans that produce the healthiest, best-tasting coffees to drink.

Once we knew that the healthiest coffees grow in high-altitude equatorial regions, we contacted the best coffee buyers and suppliers, such as Royal Coffee, Allegro, Ally, Cafe Imports, and InterAmerican, as well as scouts and local farmers, to find beans that fit our criteria so we could test them. Below is a list of countries within the targeted range that produce the healthiest, most delicious coffees in the world. In the Resources section of this book, you'll also find our recommendations for the best beans to buy, top coffee shops, and online roasters to help you always purchase better beans.

BEST COFFEE-PRODUCING COUNTRIES

ETHIOPIA produces some of the finest coffees in the world, with the fewest defects, from the best altitudes. These were the original coffees, for it was here that arabica trees originated. Most estates have excellent farming practices, processing, and packing techniques. Their natural style of dry processing dries the coffee bean within the cherry, so that they absorb wonderful blueberry taste and natural sugar. Consequently, Ethiopian coffees are characterized by light, floral, fruity notes, but they lack the fuller body and cocoa flavors of the Latin American coffees that many Americans are used to. Still, with so much flavor, Ethiopian coffees are fantastic for coffee drinkers trying to wean themselves from cream and sugar. The high CGA content gives Ethiopian coffees a carbonation-like zing, which brings their flavors to the fore. My favorite Ethiopian coffee is called Hambela. It tests better than any other coffee from Africa for taste and mouthfeel, but also has fantastic levels of polyphenols.

KENYA produces *my* favorite coffees in the world. Grown at ultrahigh altitudes, they produce top levels of CGA, bringing intense, sparkling acidity with lovely berry-like tastes. Kenyan coffees tend to have an ideal blend of fruity, East African flavor, plus more of the body traditionally found in Latin American coffees. The natural sugars are so striking than many drinkers of Kenyan coffees give up adding their own.

COLOMBIA employs some of the finest processes in Latin America devoted to providing quality coffees, including sorting machines that remove defective beans. The chief advantage of Colombian coffees is that they have the traditional body and flavor that many Americans are accustomed to, but also the big benefits of the better East African coffees. Proximity to the United States greatly reduces shipping costs and times. To me, the prize of Colombian coffee hails from the high-altitude farms in Huila.

BRAZIL produces 34 percent of the world's coffee, more than any other nation, with tremendous variation in cost and quality. In our laboratory testing, we identified big-benefit coffees with robust tastes from excellent, high-altitude farms, such as the family-owned Bobolink farms. I prefer Brazilian coffees used in blends rather than on their own. For instance, blending a Bobolink with an Ethiopian Hambela will deliver the light, fruity tones of Ethiopia as well as the body and chocolaty taste of Brazil. While Brazilian coffees are known for cheaper prices and large volumes, you can find some wonderful surprises among them if you search.

FARMING PRACTICES AND MICROENVIRONMENTS

Even within the world's best coffee-growing regions, bean quality can vary substantially from farm to farm. I learned this lesson best in Nyeri, Kenya, which is a renowned coffee district not far from the scene of my long-ago bout with altitude sickness and big game. For several years I've supported an orphanage in Kenya, and through my work there, I met Tabitha and Joshua Kagunyi, local pastors who work for the organization Feed My Starving Children. These two are remarkable in their ability to bring good to the most remote areas. Serving people in places accessible only by a series of planes and motorcycles, Tabitha and Joshua are expert local guides, and were incredibly helpful to me when I was trying to locate small coffee farms in the area.

BOB ARNOT, M.D.

Later, in the lab, our testing revealed that green beans I'd bought from neighboring estates in Nyeri varied in their levels of the chlorogenic acid 3-CQA from 32,000 milligrams per kilogram to as low as 15,000 milligrams per kilogram. The top-scoring beans, from an estate called Karogoto, held *twice* the phenol values of some Nyeri coffees. The lower scorer certainly proved far better than the supermarket beans we'd tested, which scored only 1,800 milligrams per kilogram, but still, I wanted to know what causes such a difference in beans from the same area. The quality of a farmer's practices, it turns out, and the diversity of the microenvironment he creates, have the power to transform good beans into great ones. Closer investigation revealed that the Karogoto farmers had been awarded the top prize for agricultural practices.

Having a great vine doesn't guarantee that you'll produce an award-winning wine, nor can a premium coffee plant promise a perfect cup of coffee. The best growers manipulate all the factors within their grasp, such as choosing where to plant based on sun exposure, cloud cover, and wind patterns. Because the composition and acidity of the soil affect the taste of a coffee plant's beans, other organisms planted within the same microenvironment contribute to the coffee's flavor as well. Environmental influence on flavor is known as *terroir*, a French term for the complete set of factors that nourish a fruit. Like wine aficionados, coffee lovers prefer particular terroirs because they enjoy the unique flavors generated in certain microenvironments and microclimates. My own favorite is that south-facing slope of Mt. Kenya.

My friend Barth Anderson, who cofounded Barrington Coffee Roasting Company in Massachusetts, knows a lot about terroir. I met Barth in the cupping room at Royal Coffee (an international importer in South Plainfield, New Jersey), where he was discussing his love of Ethiopian Hambela coffee, which grabbed my attention because it happens to contain huge amounts of phenols. Barth sources the coffees that Barrington roasts, and has a knack for tracking down top-notch beans from cooperatives and family farms in specific microclimates around the globe.

When variables like elevation, temperature, and rainfall are equal, it's the art of cultivation that makes some beans better from the start. Cultivating good soil is key, and the most complex soil systems, Barth says, produce the highest-quality coffees. In vast, open spaces growing nothing but coffee, the only nutritional input to the soil is from the coffee plants themselves. The simplest example of a complex system, on the other hand, is a crop planted beneath a tree canopy. The coffee plants get protective shade as well as soil enriched by the organic matter that falls from the trees. Similarly, coffees planted in volcanic soils, which are rich in minerals, produce better beans as well.

In Nyeri, the Tekangu Cooperative (of which Karogoto is a member) has won awards for some of the best farming practices in Kenya. Its farmers do an excellent job with soil cultivation, cherry sorting, and fermentation. Tekangu beans, as a result, teem with healthy phenols and win top taste scores on Coffee Review (coffeereview.com), the most widely trusted coffee review site.

CHERRY PROCESSING

A coffee bean is really a seed tucked within a cherry, which is the fruit produced by coffee plants. The sorting of cherries at harvest, fermentation, processing, and even the packaging of beans will affect the quality of the coffee they'll make. While the chief objective in packaging is to prevent beans from getting stale, cherry processing can really impact flavor.

While interviewing the Starbucks research team at their home office in Seattle, I met a man named Major Cohen, who's been with the company for twenty-one years. Once a barista and district manager, now a senior project manager, Major might be the most enthusiastic coffee fan on the planet. The joy of coffee emanates from him. Major knows just about every aspect of the coffee business inside and out, and shared with us his guidance on pairing coffees with complementary foods, which you can find in chapter 6. A surprising degree of the flavor in coffee, he told me, derives from the way the cherries are processed. "The miracle of nature plays a huge part in the taste of coffee," Major says. But so do people. "When the fruit is picked from the tree, a person has to take the fruit and skin off the seed, and the way they do that plays a huge part in how it's going to taste," he says.

There are multiple ways to process coffees; some of the methods include washed, wet-hulled, natural or dry process, and honey process. Since availability of water typically determines which method is most commonly used, the breakdown is largely geographic. Central American and South American producers (excluding Brazil) typically use the washed method. Producers in Brazil, the world's leader in arabica production, uses the natural or dry methods for the vast majority of their coffee. Coffees from Asia and the Pacific are commonly wet-hulled, and those from Africa are often processed with the natural and washed methods.

Barth tells me that processing will overwhelm origin and variety. You can take a coffee that's not fruity, for example, and make it taste fruity by processing it a certain way. From a flavor standpoint there's no good or bad way to process beans; it's purely subjective. "When well executed, they're all wonderful and different," Barth says. He likens coffee to beer in this regard. "It isn't like a pilsner, or a porter, or true ale is the only way. You can love them all."

Decaf coffee, the result of another type of processing, seems to many people a little like nonalcoholic beer, and has an equally dismal reputation for wretched taste. However, there are some excellent decaf coffees out there, full of antioxidants and scoring incredibly high marks in taste. Caffeine is removed from green coffee beans by using water, carbon dioxide, methylene chloride, or ethyl acetate as a solvent to separate and extract caffeine. (While the chemical ring of methylene chloride or ethyl acetate may trigger concern for their impact on health, they are widely regarded as safe, are approved by the FDA, and leave negligible residue on beans. Nonetheless, I recommend the water-based systems Descamex and Swiss Water Process.)

Regardless of the solvent used, decaffeinated beans become trickier to roast, which is one reason why decaf coffee often tastes bad. But I've discovered two producers who are creating amazing decaf. For me, a slow caffeine metabolizer, finding them was the best discovery I made in researching this book. The first is a group of farmers in Ethiopia who've produced a spectacular coffee from the Sidama region. Second is Mexican Natural Decaf Esmeralda, which uses the water method of extracting caffeine called Descamex. When we analyzed this coffee in the lab, the results were shocking. While the coffee contained only moderate levels of CGAs, it bore a variety of other phenols at levels we'd almost never seen in coffee. In terms of health benefits, it's ideal, with high phenols, low lipids (fats), and very little caffeine.

COFFEE SPECIES AND VARIETALS

Now that I know more about coffee, I chuckle when I see the label "100% arabica" on coffee bags. Arabica is a species of coffee plant, used in 80 percent of coffees. It's a very generic designation, like categorizing a wine simply as red. It's true, arabica beans generally are the best tasting, but unique flavors and characteristics differentiate the many varietals within the species.

Some of them have benefited from decades of natural selection. Some have storied pasts, like the Bourbon varietal, which yields a smaller harvest than most, but produces dense little cherries with excellent cup quality. Bourbon was first cultivated on an island in the Indian Ocean called Reunion, which was claimed and renamed Ile Bourbon by the king of France in the mid-1600s. Named for the island, the prized coffee was ferried by priests to Kenya, where it has thrived for over a century.

In the 1930s, the Kenyan government hired a company called Scott Laboratories to develop beans that could resist the droughts that periodically struck East Africa. One of my favorites, SL 28, failed as a high-yield coffee, but tastes extraordinarily delicious. Citric, sweet, and balanced, SL 28 coffee beans now produce some of the highest-quality coffees. Planted in south central Kenya, the bean does extremely well at high altitude. It also thrived when transplanted to Kona, Hawaii, where its coffee scored a rare 94 out of 100 points on Coffee Review.

Arabica's less popular cousin, robusta, developed an inferior reputation in Africa during colonial days, when only white settlers were permitted to grow arabica. Many price-sensitive producers today rely on the species to produce very inexpensive coffee. Drinking dark-roasted coffee masked with cream and sugar, many consumers can't tell the difference between robusta and arabica. Despite their reputation for tasting bad, robusta coffees boast two advantages. They are naturally higher in CGAs and lower in fats. For better or worse, they also contain more caffeine than arabica coffees.

PROOF: THE COFFEE CHEMISTRY LAB

"Doc!"

Raul's excited voice burst through the phone from his laboratory.

"Doc, we've found it!"

After more than a year of sourcing the most outstanding coffee beans we could find in Africa, Asia, and the Americas, and after months of testing them, Raul

Sanchez, a chemist and owner of one of the top analytical coffee chemistry facilities in the United States, saw a phenol count spike higher than he'd ever seen. "The chromatogram is off the chart!" he said. This bean was at least twice as good as any we'd tested, he told me. The phenol values were 100 percent higher than the other very good ones; they were 400 percent higher than the commercial coffees we'd tested.

We wanted to enable coffee lovers to choose the very best coffees. For taste and aroma, the Specialty Coffee Association's Q Grader course has become a widely used, uniformed approach to scoring coffees. But what about health benefits? I knew some beans were better than others. I now knew where they grew and why they were better, but I wanted quantifiable proof. After calling labs across the country and around the world, I found almost no one who would test for the biologically active components of coffee. The only research we found on the polyphenol content of coffee was being conducted by Nestlé in Switzerland. Given phenols' incredible ability to aid in weight loss, improve vascular function, reduce inflammation, lower blood sugar, and reduce blood pressure, we wanted to compare coffees based on phenol content. So we dove in, funding our own unique, comprehensive testing program to find which coffee beans, roasts, grinds, and brewing techniques would deliver the greatest number of health benefits in a cup of coffee.

BOB ARNOT, M.D.

On a country lane called Moonlight Terrace in Montpelier, Vermont, inside a quaint building that belied the sophisticated equipment it held, Raul and his team were at work measuring phenols in parts per million. Raul had become my collaborator in charting this new territory, and was as excited about it as I was. Now, after performing hundreds upon hundreds of tests utilizing high-performance liquid chromatography (HPLC), he discovered a coffee bean surging with phenols. We called it the superbean.

Raul had no idea which bean it was, as all the samples had been blinded to the chemists, but immediately I took its code, found its name, and looked it up on Coffee Review. Its staggering taste score was 94 out of 100, a score not often exceeded. In my experience, a healthy derivative of a food usually tastes like sawdust, or at least has big taste compromises. Not here. We found that high phenol levels are markers for the healthiest beans, which, in turn, offer the very best tastes.

We tested all kinds of beans. We tested those we'd acquired in our global search. We went to the largest local supermarkets and the best specialty foods stores and coffee shops to buy everything on the shelves, including Starbucks, Green Mountain, Peet's, Dunkin' Donuts, and Vermont Artisan. Online we bought Death Wish, Koffee Kult, Bulletproof, Lavazza, and many others. The laboratory bought standards for three prevalent polyphenols in coffee, called

3-, 4-, and 5-caffeoylquinic acid (CQA), which are the scientific names for specific chlorogenic acids. Using HPLC, we measured the coffees against those standards down to parts per million, and found staggering differences.

Even among the very highest-scoring green beans, 3-CQA levels ranged from 41,884 milligrams per kilogram in a Sitio Rezende to only 13,595 in a Kenyan Wachuri. In roasted beans, the differences ranged from 25,819 in a lean-roasted Ethiopian Hambela to 1,907 in a very popular high-energy coffee that is heavily roasted.

PHENOL COMPARISON AMONG WINES AND TEAS

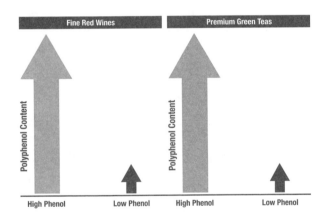

The large differences we found between high- and low-phenol coffees were also found across a range of healthy fruits and beverages. Here, a Cabernet Sauvignon and an Honest green tea are found far superior.

BOB ARNOT, M.D.

I asked experts from the Plants for Human Health Institute at North Carolina State University about these results, and learned that similar disparities have been found between the very best fruits and vegetables and the also-rans. Wild Alaskan blueberries, for instance, have significantly more polyphenols than store-bought blueberries. Scientific literature reports similarly vast differences in phenol levels of various green teas, red wines, dates, and olive oils.

We found that high-altitude Kenyan coffees routinely outscored lower altitude coffees from the Far East. We also found, with great consistency, that the beans with the highest antioxidant levels had won scores of 91 to 94 out of 100 on Coffee Review, demonstrating that you can have the very best artisanal tastes with the very highest benefits. The superbean with the score of 94 turned out to be a Kenyan Gathugu from Nyeri, which was one of the best coffees of that year. It's the best I've ever tasted.

We didn't stop at counting phenols. We tested green beans to find each coffee's maximum potential. (You probably remember the green coffee craze spurred by the powerful effects of raw coffee's antioxidants.) For each bean, we determined both the amounts of total phenols and of CGA in particular. To learn how to get the highest amount of these in a cup of coffee, we tested the effects of various roast temperatures on the phenol content. We tested grind sizes and brewing techniques to learn which ones generate the highest extraction of phenols from the grounds. Coffee has only a few potentially harmful components, such as acrylamide, and we tested for those, too.

Much of the work stands on the shoulders of generations of coffee scientists, the SCAA, and others, but bridging the data gap required complex laboratory testing using cutting-edge techniques only recently pioneered. What we ultimately found in the testing blew holes in many long-held myths about coffee. For instance, darker roasts are said to have less caffeine, but our testing showed almost no difference between caffeine content in light and dark roasts.

In the coming chapters we'll share the results of our unique lab work, to help you buy or make coffee that not only tastes great and perks you up, but also contributes to lifelong wellness.

COFFEE LAB: CGA CONTENT OF SPECIALTY AND COMMERCIALLY AVAILABLE COFFEES

As a group, specialty coffees contain considerably more chlorogenic acids than most commercially available coffees, yet they vary a good deal from each other. The following table indicates the amount of the chlorogenic acid 3-CQA found in the highest-scoring specialty coffees that we tested. Compare them to one another, but also to our corresponding chart for high-scoring commercially available coffees, some of which earned very good marks.

TOP 16 SPECIALTY COFFEES

SPECIALTY COFFEE BRAND	BENEFITS (3-CQA mg/kg)
Dr. Danger Hard Core (Extra Light)	19162
Hacienda La Minta Kenya–Nyeri AB Plus	18355
Brio Ethiopia Adado	18109
Barrington Coffee Hambela	17361
Demitasse Roasting Kenya Kii AA	16825
Daktari Coffee Kenya Nyeri Ichamama	15858
Demitasse Roasting–Congo Hutwe Ukununu	15653
Brio Mexico Chiapas	15338
Daktari Coffee Kenya Nyeri Mahiga	14875
Frequency Blend (Intelligentsia)	13335
Allegro Kenya Grand	12966
Dr. Danger Surgical Strike (Fresh)	12771
Brio Rwanda Kabirizi	12019
Three Africans–Blue Bottle	11085
Hair Bender–Stumptown Coffee Roasters	9972
Espresso Bel Canto	8729
Westrock Coffee Co. East African Blend	7021

TOP 26 COMMERCIAL COFFEES

COMMERCIAL COFFEE BRAND	BENEFITS (3-CQA mg/8-oz cup)
Dunkin' Donuts Original Blend	11042
Lavazza Kilimanjaro	8777
Bulletproof	8699
McCafe Decaf Medium Roast	8668
Starbucks Veranda Blend Blonde K-Cup	8135
Green Mountain Coffee Breakfast Blend K-Cup	8133
Colombia Luminosa (Peet's Coffee)	8033
Eight O'Clock Coffee Colombian Medium	8027
Panera Bread Light Roast	7786
Burundi Murambi New (Starbucks Reserve)	7296
Melitta Classique Supreme Medium	7247
Folgers Classic Roast	7124
Eastern D.R. Congo Lake Kivu New (Starbucks Reserve)	6990
Newman's Own Breakfast Blend	6885
Melitta Morning Bliss Light Roast	6699
Kauai Coffee Koloa Estate Medium	6592
Green Mountain Coffee Southern Pecan	6447
Maxwell House Original Roast	6227
Kicking Horse Coffee Decaf	3226
Peet's Coffee House Blend Deep Roast	2755
Peet's Major Dickason's Blend Dark	2750
Signature Select Costa Rica Medium	2277
Seattle's Best Coffee Signature Blend #3	2103
Gevalia Kaffe French Roast	2039
Starbucks Caffe Verona Dark	2026
Starbucks Verona Dark K-Cup	1968

BOB ARNOT, M.D.

That myth that dark roasts are less caffeinated than light roasts? Take a look at this chart, which shows very little difference in milligrams of caffeine at the two ends of the roast spectrum.

CAFFEINE LEVELS AND ROAST TEMPERATURE

The Coffee Lab roasted coffees in 5-degree increments, then tested them for caffeine levels. There is a very slight trend toward less caffeine as you go from a light roast on the left to a dark roast on the right.

NATURALLY HEALTHY VS. ADDITIVES OR SUPPLEMENTS

The perfect cup of coffee should contain a big load of antioxidants and anti-inflammatory compounds. Certainly, we could have added these substances into any beverage (or food or pill), but that strategy rarely works, either because the beverage, food, or pill is a poor delivery mechanism, or because the additive is not bioavailable, meaning it sails through the body instead of being absorbed. And additives affect taste as well as purity. We wanted something pure that is naturally healthy, and better beans are just that. Powerful antioxidant and anti-inflammatory compounds already are part of the bean, and a warm beverage is the ideal delivery vehicle for them.

BUYING BEANS

SINGLE ORIGIN

Buying coffee that comes from a specific microclimate or estate is one of today's hottest trends. It used to be enough for a seller to say that a coffee came from Kenya. Then buyers began to look for coffees from certain regions or towns, like Nyeri. Now aficionados are looking for beans from single estates, such as Karogoto or Gathugu. This explains the proliferation of exotic names circulating at great roasteries like Barrington, Brio, Intelligentsia, and Blue Bottle. The popularity of single-origin coffees gives specialty roasters a great opportunity to distinguish themselves from the big chains. A single estate might produce only eighty bags of beans, while a national retailer needs hundreds of thousands of bags available for a product line. In this niche, then, microroasters have a big advantage. In addition to the southwest corner of Mt. Kenya, my favorite microclimate is the Hambela region of Ethiopia. Coffee Review is a great guide to quality single-origin coffees, as are many local roasters.

BLENDS

There are three main reasons that roasters blend multiple coffees into a product: taste, cost, and benefits. Blending is a terrific way to create a greater range of tastes. Many Ethiopian coffees, for example, have that light taste that is usually described as fruity and floral but lacks the body and the chocolate, nutty flavor that many people love. I like to describe a good blend as being like a great piece of music. In this case, the Ethiopian coffee brings the high notes, which are pleasing and exciting, but need some balance. Brazilian coffees offer medium and low notes. We made a test coffee called Surgical Strike that blends Ethiopian and Brazilian beans, combining the bright high notes of East Africa with the full-bodied characteristics of South America. While single-origin coffees are popular for good reason, blending single origins, in my opinion, offers the best of both worlds.

MOCHA JAVA was the original blend, reflecting the earliest trading routes for coffee. Ships carrying coffee from Java to Europe would stop in Mocha to pick up local Yemeni coffee, then combine it with the Java. As the main port for those making the pilgrimage to Mecca, Mocha was, for a time, one of the busiest ports in the world. This time-tested blend remains one of my favorites.

For sophisticated roasters, blending is a cost-effective tool for maintaining a consistent taste profile. As costs and harvests vary throughout the year, roasters can preserve a flavor profile that's unique to a brand by substituting various beans. This is hard to do, but Starbucks, Keurig, Dunkin' Donuts, and others have mastered the technique. (Yes, Dunkin' Donuts. As the table on page 90 shows, they have terrific scores for phenols.)

The most innovative form of blending now is mixing beans with different characteristics to create a higher-benefit coffee. My English friend Robin Birley, owner of the famous nightclub 5 Hertfort Street, adds a small amount of robusta to his arabica beans to give his coffee a spike of effervescence. Nestlé has pioneered a coffee that contains some green bean to raise its phenol content. By combining beans that bring different benefits, you can architect incredible performance advantages.

COST

Hopefully, I've convinced you of the importance of buying quality coffee beans. They will deliver the health benefits that keep putting coffee in the news, like reducing the risk of diabetes, heart disease, and depression. Better beans will taste so good that you won't need to cover burnt or bitter flavors with fattening cream and sugar. And, yes, they will cost a little more.

The difference is warranted, both in terms of getting what you pay for and supporting hardworking growers who use sustainable practices. According to an international pharmacoeconomics group, coffee may be the most cost-effective way to prevent chronic illnesses.[1] Since coffee is one of the most widely consumed beverages worldwide, and numerous studies point to its ability to prevent some chronic diseases and cancers, the group ran a cost-benefit analysis that found that coffee compared favorably to other health care interventions, at lesser cost.

While you benefit from good coffee, so do its producers. Handpicking berries is an expensive and time-consuming task. But prices for coffee, a commodity crop for much of history, have remained low, even while inflation climbed for other goods. Nate Van Dusen, a brilliant roaster who cofounded Brio Coffeeworks, my favorite local roastery in Burlington, Vermont, worked in international development for years before opening his shop. Low coffee prices, he says, "have been a real problem for a lot of developing countries." When bringing better coffees to consumers, Nate adds, specialty coffee companies are asking customers to pay a higher price in order to pass on as much as possible to the coffee growers.

It's slowly beginning to work. As consumers have begun to value higher-grade coffees, their sales are bringing newfound and much-needed prosperity to small-scale growers in Africa, Asia, and the Americas. Major Cohen believes that, in this way, coffee makes the world a smaller place. This daily ritual can be for consumers "a link to parts of the world where people don't have the same benefits available as we do in the more developed world," he says. In my many visits to African nations, I've seen higher revenues from coffee sales translate to better schools and better health care. Because development in the coffee industry is more sustainable than short cycles of charitable donations, I'd love to see more promotion of good agricultural practices by governments in coffee-producing countries, allowing farmers to profit from the sale of premium coffees. In this way, perhaps, more nations could pull themselves out of poverty.

WHERE AND WHAT TO BUY

You don't have to travel the world to find great coffee beans, although it would make for a really fun trip. Look for coffees from countries near the equator, at high elevations, like

Kenya, Ethiopia, Colombia, and Brazil. If you really get sucked in, you can get to know the growing regions, the varietals, and the processing methods. A wealth of resources is accessible online, such as the Specialty Coffee Association of America, Royal Coffee, and Coffee Review, where you can check taste scores and buy beans. Putting the results of our extensive testing and coffee tasting to work for you, we've compiled our recommendations for the top five contenders among cafes to visit and online roasters to order from, as well as a list of recommended coffees, all of which can be found in the Resources section of this book. For those of you who like a shortcut, this is your ticket to better beans, and better coffee for a better life.

THE RECAP

1. Some coffee beans are much better than others!
2. Look for beans from high altitudes, near the equator, to get the highest phenol counts, the biggest benefits, and the best taste.
3. Coffee-producing countries with the biggest-benefit beans:
   Ethiopia
   Kenya
   Colombia
   Brazil

4. Go to the Resources section to see our recommendations for the top five U.S. cafés, top five sites for ordering coffee online, and a list of great-tasting high-phenol coffees.

Q AND A

Q. HOW SHOULD I STORE MY COFFEE BEANS?

A. Not in the fridge! Coffee beans are like little sponges. Roasting has made them devoid of moisture, so they'll absorb whatever they can. If you store them in the fridge and open them before they reach room temperature, moisture will form on the seeds and stale them instantaneously. A new study[2] suggests that deep freezing beans may result in more uniform particles when grinding and better taste, but you run the risk of staling if your storage isn't completely airtight. I recommend using an opaque, airtight container to store your beans at room temperature. Coffee beans are decorative and beautiful, but avoid clear canisters, which allow light to compromise the taste of your coffee. Keep your beans in a convenient, but dark and cool, location. Near the oven or stove, or on the counter in the sun, will be too warm.

Q. HOW LONG WILL MY BEANS STAY FRESH?

A. Not long, once the bag is opened. Buy beans in small quantities, such as twelve-ounce bags. Since beans begin to de-

BOB ARNOT, M.D.

grade the instant they are exposed to oxygen, it's best to buy coffee in small bags and use them within three to four days after opening. Ask for bags that are nitrogen-flushed to prevent oxidation and preserve taste for several months until opened.

Q. IS COFFEE HEALTHY FOR EVERYONE?

A. No. Caffeine-sensitive consumers may suffer ill effects from drinking too much caffeinated coffee. Slow caffeine metabolizers may experience an increase in blood pressure if they drink more than a cup or so a day. However, high-phenol decaf will provide similar benefits without risk.

Q. WHAT'S THE DIFFERENCE IN BENEFITS BETWEEN A REALLY GOOD COFFEE AND A REALLY BAD ONE?

A. Staggering. In testing how much benefit goes into your cup, we found that coffees can have as low as 6 milligrams of polyphenols. The very best we have tested has 1,096 milligrams in a cup. The low-end coffee delivers almost no benefit at all. Just one cup of the high-end coffee, however, is enough for a day, or more.

Q. WHY DO I FEEL LIKE I'M UNDERGOING DETOX WITH HIGH-POLYPHENOL COFFEES?

A. Some of our dieters say that they feel as if they are being detoxed. Why? Most of them were so inflamed from their poor diets that the incredible anti-inflammatory effects of the coffee literally make them feel as good as they have during a detox. I've learned that coffee may provide the ultimate detox since it strikes at inflammation, the key driver of so much illness from heart disease to depression.

Q. WHAT'S SO BAD ABOUT PREGROUND COFFEE?

A. One of coffee's biggest appeals is the aroma you smell when you grind beans. Soon after grinding, much of that aroma vanishes into thin air. Days or weeks later, the coffee has lost much of its flavor. With far more surface area than whole beans, ground coffee is more vulnerable to oxygen exposure, which destroys taste. (CGAs, however, are robust, and can survive grinding.)

Q. DO SOME COFFEES NATURALLY HAVE LESS CAFFEINE?

A. Yes. Caffeine acts as a natural insect repellant, so low-altitude coffees have more to combat the higher insect presence. Many of the East African coffees contain much less caffeine because they are grown at high altitude, where there are far fewer pests. A conventional coffee might have 170 milligrams of caffeine in a cup, while a Kenyan coffee could have as little as 137 milligrams per cup.

BOB ARNOT, M.D.

Q. DOES CAFFEINATED OR DECAFFEINATED COFFEE HAVE MORE BENEFIT?

A. Tricky question. We found the very best caffeinated coffees to have about 25 percent more phenols than the very best decafs. Here's the rub: With a powerful extraction process like Greek coffee has, you'll get as much as four hundred milligrams of caffeine in a single cup, and possibly more than one thousand milligrams per kilogram of phenols. To stay within the FDA guidelines for caffeine, you could have only that one cup per day; however, a high-phenol decaf may deliver eight hundred milligrams of phenols, and you could drink half a dozen cups of it to end up with more than four thousand milligrams of phenols. That's pretty extraordinary, and is exactly what I opt to do. I feel I have unlimited energy without any caffeine jitters.

CHAPTER 3

THE ROAST

Most people realize that vegetables, when overcooked, are no longer nutritious. Adding loads of salt and butter makes them downright unhealthy. But did you know that dark roasts cook the health benefits out of coffee in just the same way? It's the deep secret about the coffee that is most popular among Americans today. Superdark roasts, swirled with cream and sugar to cover their burnt-wood taste, are the coffee equivalent of soggy green beans that have been cooked all day with a fatty ham hock or slice of bacon. In either case, what could've been a nutritional asset is transformed into a major dietary liability.

If you prefer crisp, steamed veggies, and want your coffee to work *for* and not against you, then you should explore light-roasted coffees. Some coffee connoisseurs call these Nordic roasts, after the trend in Scandinavia to roast for briefer periods at lower temperatures. I like to call them lean roasts; they're lean on roast influence and can make you lean, too. Light roasts are full of flavor and nuance, from chocolate and caramel to banana and strawberry, and they are delicious enough to forgo additives. Light roasts won't taste like the coffee you may be used to, but I have faith that you can adapt. I bet you've already made similar switches in your diet, by trading overcooked vegetables for tender-crisp ones, and white bread for whole grain. In fact, I'm hoping the really dark roasts will go the way of white bread: once a favored taste, now left on the shelf for lack of nutrition.

Let me assure you, light roast doesn't mean weak coffee. Coffee becomes stronger and bolder with the addition of more coffee during the brewing process. Light, lean coffees can be extremely strong and bold if you like them that way.

DARK-ROAST NATION

Very dark-roasted coffees are largely devoid of the polyphenols that give coffee its biggest benefits. Roasting beans at ultrahigh temperatures destroys the phenols inside, and can generate higher amounts of toxic products like acrylamide, the potentially carcinogenic chemical found in French fries and potato chips. So, if they rob coffee beans of the good things and create bad things, why are dark roasts so prevalent?

America is historically a dark-roast nation. In the era of long ocean voyages on sailing ships, imported coffee sat for months in the holds of ships, exposed to brine and bilge water and growing mold. "It was pretty funky, that green coffee," says Barth Anderson, my friend and Barrington Coffee guru. "Even if a coffee was carefully grown, bad things would happen in the transport stage." What emerged on American shores required intensive roasting to destroy mildew or mold, or, at the very least, mask it. Even today, overroasting serves to disguise flawed beans and, sometimes, roasters' mistakes.

Then there's the matter of supply. Given the global demand for coffee, dark roasts are needed to normalize poor or mediocre coffee because the world simply can't produce enough of the high-caliber coffee that shines in a light roast. "There's nowhere near enough quality coffee for all those customers," Barth says.

For many people, dark roasts formed their taste memory of coffee, those early impressions that render us fond of something because it's familiar. We grew up with the dark roast. And then came the explosive growth of specialty coffee companies with signature dark brews, which solidified our collective preference for them.

For too many customers, however, drinking dark-roasted coffee means consuming more fat, sugar, and calories. As roast temperatures rise, natural sugars found in coffee are denatured. Natural flavor is destroyed and replaced with a burnt flavor. This is where coffee, which could be the healthiest thing you do for yourself, can become a terrible mistake that you repeat every day. A premium artisanal coffee has gourmet flavors that will put any milk-and-sugar drink to shame. Enjoyed on its own merit, it has zero fat, zero sugar, and negligible calories. Consider, by contrast, the crushing toll of these two drinks by two popular coffee brands.

LARGE WHITE CHOCOLATE MOCHA

580 calories

22 grams fat

15 grams saturated fat

75 grams sugar

LARGE FROZEN CAPPUCCINO

610 calories

8 grams fat

5 grams saturated fat

105 grams sugar

In just one of these drinks you're looking at two to three *days'* worth of sugar, enough calories for a small meal, and a pile of extra fat. Both of the companies that make these drinks also sell delicious coffees with impressive phenol scores. Ask for coffee from Ethiopia, Kenya, Colombia, or Brazil, and select the lightest roast offered. It'll be like choosing a glass of fine red wine over a thirty-two-ounce soda. If you're hooked on shake-like coffee drinks, we'll introduce you to some excellent alternatives in chapter 6.

COFFEE LAB: FALLING PHENOLS

After our chemists had determined the phenol content of a host of coffees, we set our sights on finding a roast that would preserve as many of these antioxidants as possible, and still taste great. To get data on the destruction of phenols during roasting, we roasted beans in ten-degree increments, then tested each sample for total phenols, and for CGAs alone.

Remember, CGA is coffee's MVP. This powerful polyphenol can quell inflammation, inhibit oxidation, lower blood sugar, and reduce blood pressure. The chart on the next page shows a top Kenyan bean's CGA content starting at 380 degrees, a benchmark known as first crack, which produces the earliest drinkable coffee. Look how quickly CGAs plummet after the roast temperature reaches 390 degrees. Their melting point is 407 degrees. A Vienna roast usually finishes above 440 degrees; a French roast,

EFFECT OF ROASTING ON CHLOROGENIC ACID (3-CQA)

IN A TOP KENYAN BEAN

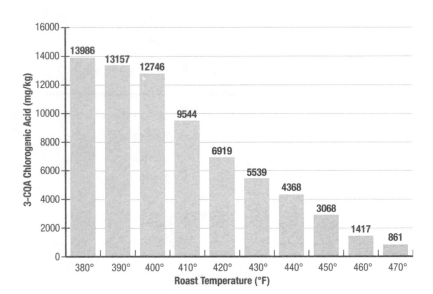

This graph shows the decline in a key chlorogenic acid (3-CQA) as roast temperature increases. You can see the tremendous concentrations in very light roasts to the left. However only 6 percent of the cga remains in the darkest roast to the right.

BOB ARNOT, M.D.

above 460 degrees. In this bean, CGAs bottomed out before we even reached those temperatures. At the finish of roasts we tested, light roasts had lost 30 percent of CGAs, medium roasts had lost 50 percent, and dark roasts nearly 90 percent.

The chart on page 110, depicting total phenols at ten-degree increments in the same bean, tells a less dramatic story. The phenols fall, but they don't crash. This is because CGA gets transformed into other phenols and antioxidants as the roast temperature rises. One of these compounds is a melanoidin that's created in the medium-roast stage and can be helpful in the gut, offering protection from fatty meals. Because different polyphenols develop as roasts progress, some roasters say there remains value in dark roasts, but as the temperature soars, even the melanoidins drop off sharply. The highest total antioxidant capacity is found in light to medium roasts, as was also shown in a study at the University of Zurich's famous coffee lab.[1] For a coffee to emerge from a dark roast with an effective level of phenols is highly unlikely, and requires starting with an incredibly good green bean that is ultrahigh in CGA.

I created the temperature scale on page 111 to help you put some commonly used roast names together with finish temperatures, and see our corresponding CGA counts.

Beyond the medium roasts, the coffees' natural flavors are eclipsed by those of the roast. Also at that point, our lab work showed that CGA is in sharp decline. You can enjoy a darker roast with a roast temperature just over 430 degrees; it's the truly burnt coffees finished above 470 degrees that have little value left. Those coffees are in no way dangerous, but you'll miss out on the many benefits and taste delights of a lighter roast. If you really love dark roasts, there are superb ones from companies like Peet's that will still

TOTAL PHENOLS AND ROAST TEMPERATURE

The Coffee Lab tested beans for complete polyphenol content. With increasing temperature, polyphenols diminished, however less so than with our test for chlorogenic acids. The test shows there are still substantial amounts of polyphenols in medium roasts.

BOB ARNOT, M.D.

benefit you. Ask for a city roast or full city roast, which will still have some phenolic value, since Peet's starts out with great beans.

WHAT HAPPENS AS HEAT IN THE ROASTER RISES

- **380 DEGREES:** First crack, when a bean begins to break open. Coffee cupped here will taste thin and grassy. Total CGAs: 51,234.
- **385: CINNAMON ROAST.** Sharply acidic, taste still underdeveloped.
- **390:** CGA remains high, although coffee is not fully developed by most standards. Total CGAs: 46,475. The very best roasters can create a lean roast here with tremendous benefits and good taste using premium Kenyan and Ethiopian coffees.
- **400: LEAN ROAST.** Sugars begin to develop, bringing sweetness and flavor. Total CGAs: 44,354. Good specialty roasters can nail a great taste at this temperature through 405.
- **405: LIGHT ROAST.** Effervescent cup of coffee. This is the beginning of the sweet spot for many East African coffees.
- **410: AMERICAN ROAST.** Robust, good flavor. Total CGAs: 32,804. In our testing, CGA is being destroyed at this temperature, but is rapidly replaced with other antioxidants. Good compromise roast for maintaining original flavors and benefits. The bean appears light brown.

- **415: MEDIUM ROAST.** Sweet spot for many South American coffees.
- **420:** Sugars begin to caramelize. Robust flavors for many Latin American coffees. Total CGAs: 24,926.
- **428–430: CITY ROAST.** Begin to taste the roast, but natural flavors still punch through. Total CGAs: 19,567.
- **437: FULL CITY ROAST.** Medium dark. This is the beginning of the second crack. Total CGAs: 13,829.
- **440–450: VIENNA ROAST.** Little trace of the original taste of the bean itself left. Total CGAs: 9,282.
- **464: FRENCH ROAST.** The coffee has a noticeably burnt taste. Intrinsic flavors of the bean have been eliminated. This is the end of the second crack. Total CGAs: 4,912.
- **473: ITALIAN ROAST.** Burnt tones become quite noticeable. Acidity and body significantly reduced. Total CGAs: 2,972.

INTO THE LIGHT

If you're going to invest in good beans, consider leaving the Dark-Roast Nation behind, and choose a light or medium roast that will preserve their natural flavor and antioxidant value. Remember that CGA, with all its anti-inflammatory, disease-fighting power, begins a sharp decline when roast temperatures reach about 390 degrees and, after that, it's in free fall. At 430 degrees, 75 percent of CGA is gone.

Making the switch may take some getting used to, as many coffee drinkers have grown so accustomed to the burnt flavor of dark roasts that they perceive it to be the taste of good coffee. "What people interpret as quality," says Barth, "is roast forward. Meanwhile, there are these coffees that are the *grand crus* of coffee experience yielding a whole other realm of aroma and taste, where roast takes quite a backseat."

That vast realm is depicted in a new flavor wheel, created in 2016 by the Specialty Coffee Association of America and the World Coffee Research Sensory Lexicon, which you can find at http://www.scaa.org/?page=resources&d=scaa-flavor -wheel. An update on the 1995 original, the wheel is the product of collaboration between sensory experts, scientists, coffee buyers, and roasting companies to give coffee professionals and enthusiasts a vocabulary that ensures they're talking apples to apples—or cherries to cherries.

Coffee has more than one hundred distinct flavors, which hint at fruits, flowers, nuts, spices, and even greens and woods. Light roasts, by showcasing those flavors, can top the complexities of the finest wines. In fact, the specialty coffee industry now looks much like the world of wine, with coffee sommeliers, tastings, and celebrated terroirs and estates. Specialty or third-wave roasters, those who approach coffee as an artisanal product, rather than a commodity, tend to favor lighter roasts for their ability to let unique coffees shine. "In roasting we're looking to use the lightest hand we possibly can to preserve all those nuances that are in there," says Barth. "Overroast, and you wipe out all that. You normalize coffee by roasting at too high an end temperature."

As I've mentioned, a light roast doesn't mean weak coffee. Many people mistake the term *bold* for *dark*. You can have a bold coffee, which simply means a higher ratio of coffee to water, without using dark-roasted beans. In a bold, light roast you can taste the coffee's inherent flavor, making it possible to skip the add-ons you needed to balance your dark roast. I sent a favorite light roast to my friend, Washington, DC, author, commentator, and radio host Tom Basile, who wrote this to me in return: "Bob, my wife and I were talking about your coffee—the fruity notes mean that you use less creamer and sugar, improving the health benefits of the coffee. Anyway, we love the coffee."

Tom makes a vital point. When a great roast brings out the natural flavors of a coffee, you don't have to load it up with milk and sweeteners. The mission of many specialty coffee roasters is to sell the cream-and-sugar set on the staggering world of amazing flavors that can be unlocked from within good beans.

Millennials are among those already converted. While only 9 percent of Americans currently drink light-roasted coffee, according to the National Coffee Association, 19 percent of millennials prefer light roasts. Often health-conscious and open-minded, they're leading the trend in favoring light roasts for their health and flavor superiority.

COFFEE LAB: YIKES, ACRYLAMIDE!

Acrylamide, a chemical formed when substances containing carbohydrates are roasted or heated to high temperatures, has been shown to cause cancer in animals and is classified as a possible human carcinogen. The coffee world has begun to buzz a bit about acrylamide, and some conflicting reports and advice have surfaced. While some European researchers have published reports that light-roasted coffee beans contain more acrylamide than dark-roasted beans, our lab testing concluded the opposite. In our tests, the darker the roast became, the higher acrylamide levels rose. The top chart on the next page tracks a Colombian Huila bean from 380 degrees to 470 degrees, about the temperature of an Italian roast. Acrylamide levels start at 4,311 parts per billion, and soar to a high of 14,428. To me, this is another reason to choose a lighter roast. The bottom chart on the next page depicts varying levels of acrylamide in specific coffees that we tested. Go for lower acrylamide, but do find reassurance in that hundreds of studies observe that coffee doesn't cause most cancers; it prevents them.

ACRYLAMIDE LEVELS DURING ROASTING

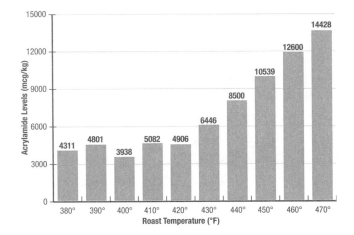

The Coffee Lab roasted coffee from very light to quite dark. As the roast temperature increased, the amount of acrylamides more than tripled. The lighter roasts have the fewest acyrlamides.

ACRYLAMIDES IN INDIVIDUAL COFFEES

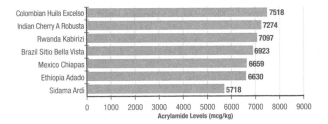

We tested these eight coffees for acrylamides. All were within a reasonable range. The lighter roasted Adado and Ardi had the lowest levels.

BOB ARNOT, M.D.

COFFEE LAB: THE REAL DEAL ON COFFEE AND ACID

Coffee is commonly believed to be acidic, but this is less true than you may think. Take a look at this chart showing acidity of several beverages we tested. (In case you haven't had to consider pH since high school chemistry class, here's a refresher: pH is the measure of acidity and basicity on a scale of zero to fourteen, in which zero is highly acidic, seven is neutral, and fourteen is strongly basic, or alkaline.) You may be surprised to see that the pH of the coffees hover around five—less acidic than most beverages, including soda, sports drinks, and apple juice!

There are several popular misconceptions on the subject of acid that I'd like to clear up. First, don't let the term *chlorogenic acid* mislead you. Many people hear the word *acid* and think: danger. But there are many types of acid out there, and the chlorogenic acids I've been extolling are light acids that give fresh coffee its effervescence and zing, and have beneficial, anti-inflammatory, and antioxidant properties. Coffees high in CGA were not more acidic in terms of pH than those with less CGA in our laboratory measurements.

Second, caffeine is in part to blame for the perception that coffee is very acidic because caffeine stimulates production of the gastric acid we know as stomach acid. If you feel your stomach churning and burning after drinking coffee, the culprit is probably not acid in your coffee, but acid

ACIDITY OF BEVERAGES

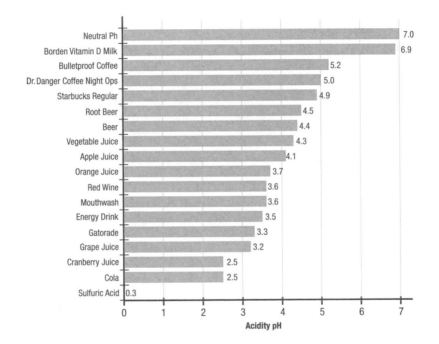

This comparison of beverages shows the range of acidity. On this scale, colas, grape juice, red wine, and beer are all far more acidic than coffee.

that caffeine has caused your body to produce. If you have problems with stomach acid, limit your caffeinated coffee and enjoy more decaf.

Last, you may have heard that dark-roasted coffee is less acidic than light-roasted, and I'm delighted to debunk that myth with good science. Technically, it is true, but it's not the whole story. When we tested high-CGA coffees in the lab, we found that, as roasting progressed, benign and helpful chlorogenic acids were transformed or destroyed, and much stronger acids, like citric, malic, and phosphoric acids, appeared. The strong acids decline significantly only in extremely dark roasts that are cooked beyond a point at which most people would drink them.

As the above chart on the next page shows, a green coffee bean has a pH of five to five and a half. The pH dips (acidity rises) briefly as roasting begins, then climbs back, as acids break up or evaporate. At the finish of a light or medium roast, the pH is between five and six, less acidic than the green bean, and fairly close to neutral seven. Only at extremely high temperatures that create undrinkable coffees does pH climb above six.

And following are two more charts showing pH levels of some specialty coffees we roasted. You can see that the pH of most is around five—less acidic than many sodas, fruit juices, and sports drinks.

EFFECT OF ROAST TEMPERATURE ON ACIDITY

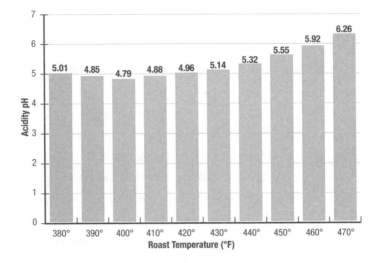

We roasted coffee from very light to quite dark. The lighter roasts were slightly more acidic. Very dark roasts were the least acidic.

COFFEE ROASTS AND ACIDITY

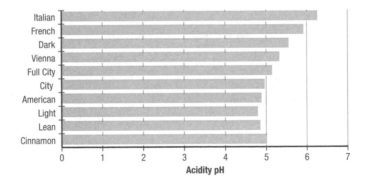

From very lean roasts to the darkest Italian and French roasts, there was a steady decline in acidity, demonstrating that very dark roasts are less acidic.

BOB ARNOT, M.D.

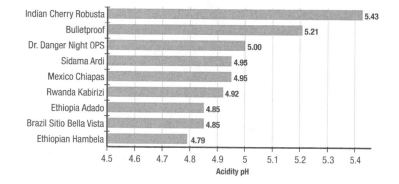

ACIDITY OF COFFEES

Coffee	Acidity pH
Indian Cherry Robusta	5.43
Bulletproof	5.21
Dr. Danger Night OPS	5.00
Sidama Ardi	4.95
Mexico Chiapas	4.95
Rwanda Kabirizi	4.92
Ethiopia Adado	4.85
Brazil Sitio Bella Vista	4.85
Ethiopian Hambela	4.79

Acidity pH

We compared coffees and found a range—from quite acidic in the Ethiopian Hambela to far less acidic in the bulletproof. Bulletproof also tested completely mycotoxin free.

"There is no significant relationship between coffee consumption and the four major acid-related upper gastrointestinal disorders."[2]

So concluded a study run by a group of Japanese scientists in 2013 to evaluate the effect of coffee on acid-related diseases. With more than eight thousand healthy adults participating, the scientists found no association between coffee consumption and the most common upper gastrointestinal diseases: gastric ulcer, duodenal ulcer, reflux esophagitis, and nonerosive reflux disease.

NOTE: If you do have reflux esophagitis, a large volume of any hot liquid could make your symptoms worse. Since this condition can lead to esophageal cancer, make sure your doctor has you on the proper medications to cut the acidity of your stomach contents.

MYTH

Coffee is bad for me because it's too acidic.

TRUTH

1. Coffee is less acidic than most sports drinks.
2. Caffeine stimulates production of gastric (stomach) acid.
3. Only extremely dark roasts are notably less acidic.

THE ART OF ROASTING

Like cooking, coffee roasting is both a science and an art. And, like great chefs, the best roasters I know cringe at the thought of overcooking. Leaving the Dark-Roast Nation to the masses, these skilled roasters tend to load heat into the roaster quickly, then get the beans out before their essential goodness is destroyed. Artful roasting will unlock the health benefits and gourmet flavors inherent in good coffee beans by drawing out sugars, fats, aromas, and phenols, while underroasting creates a thin, grassy flavor that lacks sweetness. Overroasting, as you now know, makes the coffee—well, just burnt.

Trickier than it may sound, achieving an excellent roast requires a delicate balance between preserving the components that make a coffee great and the destructive forces of the heat needed to bring them out. "We're creating a cascade of billions of chemical reactions, starting with the 1,000 or so chemicals in green coffee," says Scott Rao, a renowned coffee expert, master roaster, and author of *The Coffee Roaster's Companion* and *The Professional Barista's Handbook*. "We are constantly creating new chemicals and combinations." Adding challenge to an already complicated process, every batch of beans is different, brought to its highest potential by a different finish temperature and roast profile. "The first step in the process is to figure out what finish roast temperature is going to yield the best result," says Nate Van Dusen,

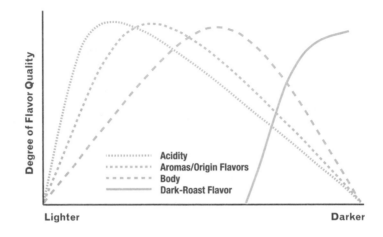

FLAVOR EMPHASIS BY ROAST DEGREE

Degree of Flavor Quality

Lighter

Darker

.... Acidity
· · · · · · · Aromas/Origin Flavors
– – – – – Body
——— Dark-Roast Flavor

This chart from coffee analysts shows how aroma and body develop as coffee is roasted. The maximum taste benefit is achieved early in the roast cycle with excellent body and aroma developed in the light to medium roasts. These natural flavors are replaced by the taste of the roast itself in the darker roasts. For high-phenol coffee, the key is to roast enough for great flavor but not so much as to destroy phenol content.

my go-to roaster in Burlington, Vermont. So, for each new batch of beans, specialty roasters run a temperature study, roasting to a finish temperature suspected to be on the outer end of what will taste best. This is a gross simplification, but gives an indication of the complexities of roasting. Samples are pulled and cupped (the coffee pros' term for controlled tasting) every five degrees or so, until they hit the sweet spot.

If you think of a finish temperature as a destination, the

roast profile is the path the roaster takes to get there. Depicted by a curve that climbs the axes of time and temperature, the roast profile can be somewhat flat, which is like a slow bake, or shoot up (shorter time, higher heat), which is like searing. If you have any experience cooking or baking, you'll know that time and temperature really influence flavor. Roast too fast and the beans scorch; roast too slow and they dry out . . . You get the picture. Nailing the timing is key. "Ten seconds one way or the other and it's a different coffee," says Barth. "It can be entirely dashed against the rocks if it's done poorly. At every point, there's a really great chance for things to go wrong."

PURSUING A PERFECT ROAST

The more I learned about roasting, the clearer it became that getting the roast right was as imperative to my quest for the perfect coffee as finding the best beans. What was one without the other? Comb the planet for coffee beans full of health benefits, and then cook them to death? Perfect a light-roast profile for a bean that held nothing worth saving? There'd be no point. Most specialty roasters focus on flavor; they want to draw out the natural sweetness in a coffee, its fruity or floral or nutty flavors. I wanted that, too, but I also wanted phenols.

So, with superb roasters from Brio Coffeeworks in Burlington, Vermont, and Excellent Coffee Company in Pawtucket, Rhode Island, who employed two veterans from George Howell Coffee (Howell is one of my ultimate coffee idols, a coffee pioneer since the 1970s and winner of international accolades), we worked to develop a perfect roast for our best beans.

This turned out to be the biggest thrill for me. At the helm of a German coffee roaster called a Probat Burns, whose control panel resembles the cockpit of a fighter jet, I learned to operate software to control the curve of the roast profile. I could carefully control the heat input during the roast to generate tremendous flavors and preserve as many polyphenols as possible. We roasted our best beans in ten-degree increments, then measured for CGA and other phenols, and cupped every sample. We wanted to be certain the coffee was pure, too, so we tested to see that it was free of pesticides and toxins. We carefully customized a roast curve that got the flavors just right, while keeping the temperature low enough to preserve polyphenols and other biologically active compounds. We wanted to roast the outsides of the beans to develop flavors and aromas, while more lightly roasting the beneficial contents of the interiors.

I was gathering knowledge about coffee's potential to improve health in the same way I've studied many subjects during my career: infectious disease, breast cancer, aging, nutrition, and others. I've come to think of myself as a knowledge engineer; I like to take complex information and put it into a form that's useful, from books to television programs, documentaries, lectures, and diets. This time, it became apparent that preparing the perfect cup of coffee is really complex. (In fact, at UC Davis there's a semester-long chemical engineering course titled "The Design of Coffee."[3]) I had studied thousands of articles from the National Library of Medical Science. I had searched the planet for the perfect coffee varietal, terroir, washing technique, and preparation. Now, I had customized a lean roast for maximum phenol content and run exhaustive laboratory testing on nearly every component of coffee.

I was eager to share the unique results of this work: charts, graphs, lists of recommended coffee-growing countries, roasters, and beans. Yet the most critical factor remained untested—taste. Many of the coffees with the highest phenol levels had scored remarkably well among the pros at Coffee Review, but we wanted regular consumers to test the coffees that we'd selected and roasted expressly for maximum phenol content. After all, no matter how healthy high-phenol coffee may be, people won't drink it if they don't think it tastes good. As part of a broader food-tech platform called Epic Harvest, we developed several sample coffee brands to test among consumers. Dr. Danger was a high-performance brand targeted for the athlete and performance-coffee customer; Daktari was a purely artisanal brand; and Phenomonol Coffee highlighted the health benefits of phenols for the general population.

Sold through Amazon, the coffees garnered exceptional feedback on flavor. Daktari won amazing scores on Coffee Review, including a highly sought 94. Customers, athletes, and dieters not only approved of the taste of the high-phenol coffees, they reported improvements in mood and vigor that mirrored those detected by the POMS instrument in our clinical trials.

CHOOSING A ROASTER

Choosing a great roaster is paramount to getting a great cup of coffee with actual benefits. You want a roaster who sources better beans and knows how to save them from the scorching of dark roasts. As you read in chapter 2, many excellent roasting companies sell online, making it possible to get some of the world's greatest coffees at your doorstep in a matter of days. The best roasters keep abreast of crops at family coffee farms and co-ops around the globe; they test roast each batch of beans; they have quality packaging and can roast to order. Coffee Review, Intelligentsia, Barrington Coffee Roasting Company in Lee, Massachusetts, which Barth cofounded with Gregg Charbonneau, and of course, our own roasting operation for test brands Dr. Danger and Daktari are among my favorites.

Even if you find a coffee you love that's available online,

it's always wonderful to discover a good local roaster. Local roasters are incredibly passionate about coffee and you may find your very best cup of coffee close to home. Plus, the beans you buy from a local roaster will likely be fresher than any others, and freshness is a total game changer. If you've been happily buying preground coffee from the grocery store, you're going to be stunned by how much better your coffee can taste. And it will be better for you. One July day in the Coffee Lab, we roasted a spectacular Kenyan Karogoto and tested it for phenols. We ran the test again six weeks later. Already, the bean had lost 20 percent of its antioxidant capabilities, and tasted pretty stale.

Nate and Magda Van Dusen, who run my favorite local roastery, Brio Coffeeworks in Burlington, Vermont, purchase top-quality beans, and coax the best out of them by meticulously test roasting to find the ideal roast profile and temperature for each batch. Nate's a stickler for freshness, so coffee from my local roaster is never stale. "Coffee is at its peak flavor a couple days to two weeks off roast," Nate says.

Find a roaster close to where you live, so you can buy something really fresh within that window. If you hang out and chat with the roaster, you can learn a great deal while you're at it. Buy small, twelve-ounce bags of beans and use them right away.

Another bit of advice from Nate: "Never buy a coffee that doesn't have a roast date on it." Many commercial roasters label coffee bags with expiration dates instead of roast dates. "Sometimes [the expiration] is nine months or a year out," he says, "which is nine months to a year past when you should buy it."

WHAT TO LOOK FOR

How do you know whether a local roasting company is a good one? First and foremost, I gauge a roaster's ability on his or her skill in producing a light roast. These are hard to perfect, and many roasters use darker roasts to cover up their sins. Even if you don't drink lighter roasts, test one to see if you can taste actual flavors. If you pick up delicate floral and fruity notes, they got it right. Next, if the company is big enough, look for their scores on coffeereview.com. Scores over 90 are hard to achieve and indicate outstanding effort. Also, talk with the roaster. He or she should be able to discuss with ease all the fine points you've encountered in this chapter, and ideally should have a tremendous interest in and zeal for producing the perfect cup. He or she should offer great bean selection and show an understanding of the microenvironments that produce high-caliber coffees. For instance, if I saw an Ichamama from Nyeri, Kenya, I'd be very impressed. If the roaster has blends and cute names, but no single-origin special reserves, I'd look elsewhere.

Remember, 90 percent of coffee is sold on pure marketing—a great name and packaging. In my area, there is a local roaster with an amazing facility, great packaging, and an epic name. But this is the review that a top coffee taster gave the company's coffee: "A foul-smelling and tasting coffee dominated by notes of petroleum, wet paper, burnt wood, and rubbery chocolate. Very dark-roasted, probably poor-quality green coffees." Because so many coffee drinkers use coffee as a carrier for cream and sugar, they don't notice when the coffee itself tastes awful!

HOW TO JUDGE A COFFEE ROASTER

1. Try a light roast. Look for delicate fruity, floral notes.
2. Look for scores on coffeereview.com.
3. Don't fall for fancy marketing and packaging.
4. Look for great bean selection and knowledge about microenvironment.
5. Look for single-origin special reserve coffees.

DON'T DISCOUNT THE BAG!

Oxygen is the great enemy of roasted coffee beans, so good packaging is critical to freshness. Bags that have a one-way valve for oxygen to escape help prevent staling, which isn't just the loss of freshness, but also the formation of off flavors. Even better is a foil bag that's nitrogen-flushed. Flushing the oxygen out of a foil bag with nitrogen preserves the taste and health benefits of your coffee longest. Ask your online or local roaster if they have them.

In the lab, we were surprised how many bags we tested had oxygen levels as high as 19 percent. The industry standard is less than 3 percent, although some coffees we tested had only 0.2 percent. (These use new oxygen scavengers, which soak up nearly every trace of oxygen.) The table on the opposite page indicates the amount of oxygen in bags of specialty and commercial coffees that we tested. The bottom line is that with significant oxygen in the bag, any coffee you buy could be stale after just a month or so, yet may have an expiration date of eighteen months from the date of roasting.

In canvassing grocery stores, we found many products with high oxygen levels nearing their expiration date. Our lab tested for a series of seven staling chemicals and found extremely high levels of staling in these older coffees with high oxygen levels. The taste experience could at best be described as poor and at worst as rancid! After all the effort roasters put into sourcing and roasting coffee, be sure that the packaging has a one-way valve, that the oxygen is below 3 percent, and that the roast date is within several months of your purchase.

OXYGEN LEVELS IN BAGS OF TESTED COFFEES

COFFEE	OXYGEN LEVEL (%)
Lavazza	0.1
Dunkin' Donuts	0.2
Gevalia	0.2
Kauai	0.2
Melitta	0.2
New England Coffee	0.2
Newman's Own	0.2
Panera	0.2
Seattle's Best	0.2
Starbucks	0.2
Daktari	3.0
Dr. Danger	3.0
Green Mountain	7.5
Signature Select	7.5
East African	8.3
McCafe	11.6
Eight O'Clock	19.4
Rockin' & Roastin'	20.6
Vermont Coffee	20.6

HOW TO STORE COFFEE

Fruits and vegetables let you know when they're old. Slimy lettuce, yellow broccoli crowns, brown, mushy bananas, weird things growing out of potatoes . . . Coffee beans do you no such favor. Every day after roasting, taste comes off the beans. Phenols decline. Yet, still, they look like classy little gems, hard and brown and smooth. Don't be deceived, however; old beans will have lost their benefits, much of their flavor, and their zing, which is why we recommend buying small bags and using them within three to four days of opening. Remember, moisture and oxygen are the enemies of great coffee.

DOS AND DON'TS FOR COFFEE STORAGE

Protect your coffee from moisture, air, and light, all of which will degrade them quickly. Here's how:

- Don't store your coffee in the refrigerator!
- Don't store preground coffee! Buy whole beans and grind before brewing.
- Do store your coffee in a cool, dry place, like a pantry.
- Do store your coffee in an airtight, opaque container.

Choosing a healthy roast is just as critical as selecting premium coffee beans. Hopefully you've begun to see those inky dark roasts in a new light, since overroasting destroys phenols and flavors, denatures sugars, creates acrylamides, and leads to major dietary mistakes. If you need to lose a good deal of weight, ditching high-fat, high-calorie, sugary coffee drinks is the perfect place to start. If you need to shed only a few stubborn pounds, cutting out half-and-half and a few spoonfuls of sugar may well do the trick. Light to medium roasts, which preserve coffee's anti-inflammatory, antioxidant powers, offer an incredible array of natural flavors, from chocolate to nutty, floral to fruity. They can serve as a gourmet taste treat with no fat or sugar, providing fuel for your workout, your workday, and your life.

THE RECAP

1. Downfalls of the dark roast:
   - Like overcooked vegetables, very dark-roasted coffee is no longer beneficial to your health.
   - Dark roasts lead many coffee drinkers to pad their diets with extra fat and sugar.
   - Dark roasts steal the spotlight. Premium coffees have all the flavor complexity and nuance of fine wines, but in a dark roast, you'll taste mainly the roast.
   - The darker the roast, the more acrylamide there may be in your coffee.
2. Light roasts offer nuanced, natural flavors.
3. Light roasts help protect your health.
4. Light roasts keep you lean!
5. Buy small, twelve-ounce bags of beans and use them right away.

6. If you order online, look for roasters who roast to order and ship within a couple of days.

7. Look for coffees with roast dates, rather than expiration dates.

8. Look for nitrogen-flushed bags with one-way valves to allow oxygen to escape; otherwise, your coffee will stale quickly.

Q AND A

Q. WHAT IF I'M A DIE-HARD DARK ROAST FAN?

A. I have several suggestions. Figure out what you like about it. If it's the taste of burnt wood, try a cupping session at a local roaster to find some other flavors that you like. There are more than 100, from blueberry to chocolate. Second, choose a light dark roast! Seriously. Roast temperatures of 450 degrees and higher nearly incinerate the polyphenols in coffee. However, a roast that finishes at 430 degrees still gives you a dark-roast taste and a decent amount of phenols. Third, it's even more important for you to look for really good beans that contain a high level of phenols when green (before the roast). Finally, roasters can singe the outside of the bean so that it tastes burnt, but leave the interior still full of phenols. Ask a local roaster if they can do this for you!

BOB ARNOT, M.D.

Q. DO DARKER ROASTS HAVE ANY ADVANTAGES?

A. Yes, their chief advantage is the production of melanoidin, which provides a strong anti-inflammatory influence and works in the large intestine to help deflect fats from being absorbed. Melanoidins reach their highest level at a medium roast, then decline as the roast becomes darker.

Q. I'VE HEARD OF THE LEAN OR FIT ROASTS FROM SCANDINAVIA. WHAT ARE THOSE?

A. Light roasts generally finish between 400 and 408 degrees. However, an extremely light roast may be as low as 380 de grees. They'll lose some taste, but have sky-high phenols. It's a big craze that is catching on abroad.

Q. IS KNOWING THE FINISHING ROAST TEMPERATURE ENOUGH TO DETERMINE WHETHER A COFFEE IS WELL ROASTED?

A. No. Roast profiles are a true art. A roaster could keep a low temperature but bake the coffee by leaving it in too long. For our test coffee brands, we look at a curve on a computer to get just exactly the shape we want. There are many different ways of getting to a final temperature, which have dramatic impacts on taste and phenols. This is why you want to choose a top roaster.

Q. HOW CAN I TELL WHO THE GREAT ROASTERS ARE?

A. Look at our list of recommended artisan specialty coffees in the Resources section. The roasters listed alongside them have both great taste scores and kill it when it comes to high phenols. Also rely on Coffee Review. They run independent taste tests. You can bet that roasters who earn scores in the nineties are fantastic. Also, check out coffeechemlab.com for the latest top-scoring coffees. You'll find test scores on popular brands for caffeine, acrylamides, polyphenols, and lots more.

Q. WHAT CAN I TELL ABOUT A ROAST BY LOOKING AT BEANS?

A. Look at the color. The lighter the color, the lighter the roast. You can also break a bean in half and look at the inside. It should be lighter than the outside. Otherwise, the bean is baked, which ruins the taste and phenol level.

Q. I NOTICE THAT MY LIGHT-ROASTED COFFEE IS VERY HARD TO GRIND. ANY SUGGESTIONS?

A. Sure. I have a very high-end Mahlkönig EK 43 grinder, and it can grind a very lightly roasted bean for only forty-five seconds before the fuse blows! Lightly roasted beans are really hard. You can try a hand grinder, but I have even broken those. Specialized espresso or Turkish grinders work well, as do inexpensive Cuisinart blenders, even though they are blade grinders. (Conical grinders produce more uniform particles, which improves taste and phenol extraction.)

Q. AT WHAT TEMPERATURE DO PHENOLS BEGIN TO BE DESTROYED?

A. On roast curves we see a slight increase in phenols from 380 to 390 degrees. Beginning at 400 degrees, the decline begins. The boiling point of CGA is between 405 and 408 degrees, so that is where the very biggest drop in CGAs occurs. Between 405 and 412 degrees, you get the very best flavors.

Q. DO BEANS DIFFER IN THEIR BEST ROAST TEMPERATURES?

A. Yes, dramatically so. Where a Kenyan coffee may taste great in the hands of a master roaster, finishing at 382 degrees, a Colombian Huila or Brazilian Bobolink may not taste great until it reaches 418 degrees.

Q. ARE SOME BEANS MORE RESISTANT TO THE DESTRUCTION OF PHENOLS?

A. Yes. In our laboratory we found the high-altitude Kenyan and Ethiopian beans to be highly resistant to degradation, whereas Latin American beans are much more vulnerable to the loss of phenols with heat.

CHAPTER 4

THE BREW

A hh . . . those fantastic aromas wafting off the head of an elegant pour-over. The final process in coffee preparation, the one that puts a warm, fragrant cup in your hands, is not just the simple ritual that most of us call brewing coffee—it's a complex feat of chemical engineering. While writing this book, I wanted to master every aspect of creating the world's best cup of coffee. So, between visiting farms high on Mt. Kenya, learning to operate the Probat Burns roaster, and poring over books on the chemical engineering of coffee, I practiced every method of brewing coffee, from the simplest to the most complex. If you're among the 73 percent of Americans who prepare their coffee at home, you can learn from some of my mistakes.

I'm a fan of aviation, and there's an analogy here with coffee, though the stakes aren't nearly as high. Pilots fly aircraft inside what is called a flight envelope, which governs speed, altitude, dives, and maneuvers to ensure that planes don't stall and crash, or break apart. I learned that coffee also has a performance envelope within which it excels, delivering spectacular benefits and incredible tastes. Push the envelope, and your cup of coffee will be ruined by becoming too sour, bitter, or burnt.

We've worked hard in the laboratory to determine exactly how to adjust each variable in all the most popular brewing techniques to find that sweet spot for coffee. We were among the first to take a two-pronged approach to testing brewing techniques, not only for the best taste profiles, but also for the greatest health benefits. The abundance of choices in how to brew coffee can be overwhelming, but fear not. In this chapter you'll learn which techniques are best at extracting healthy phenols, and how to make the most delicious coffee, whichever method you choose. Even if you don't prepare your own coffee, understanding the world of pour-over coffees when you walk into a coffee shop will vastly improve your experience.

First, set aside for now the automated devices like Keurigs and Cuisinarts. Get ready for a bit of a mess, and summon some patience. It took me a month to make a decent cup of coffee. I scalded myself a few times, and spilled hot grounds all over my kitchen counter and several friends. My worst blunder occurred at the Sloane Club in London, when I exploded an AeroPress, spilling coffee all over the rug. The bill was not cheap! So, be careful and be patient. If you don't currently prepare your own coffee, the techniques described in this chapter will seem labor intensive and time consuming. Invest time on a weekend to practice preparing your coffee. Soon, you'll be quick and efficient at making amazing coffee that can help you lose weight, perform better, and live longer.

EXTRACTION

About half of a roasted coffee bean is soluble in water. Hot water dissolves the soluble components, some of which are delicious, some healthy, some bitter, and some bad for you. Scientists call this extraction. By adjusting four key variables, you can extract all the most delicious and helpful sugars, fats, gases, and phenols, leaving behind as much as you can of the undesirable elements, like strong acids and bits of the cellulose wall of the bean, which destroy the taste of coffee.

How much of the soluble coffee should you extract to make an amazing cup of coffee? Only scientists could turn something as pleasurable as coffee into a dry examination of particles and percentages, but this is valuable intel to anyone who wants to move beyond his or her Keurig or Mr. Coffee machine. Optimal extraction balances the percentage of solubles dissolved and their concentration. The sweet spot, the very best coffee one can make, is neither too strong nor too weak, and extracts enough from the beans to produce full flavor, but no bitter components. The Specialty Coffee Association of America has pinpointed the optimal range of extraction as between 18 and 22 percent of the soluble beans.

VARIABLES

How do you control extraction? If you think of brewing coffee as a science experiment, four variables will affect your outcome, which, ultimately, is the taste and healthfulness of your coffee. They are time, water temperature, grind size, and coffee-to-water ratio. Let's take a look at how each variable affects the quality of your cup of coffee.

1. TIME: Coffee brewed too briefly will be underdeveloped, while coffee brewed too long will contain unwanted ingredients like acids, fats, and cellulose. Using a timer is important to getting your brew just right. Notice that each technique has a different ideal brew time.

IDEAL BREW TIMES
- AeroPress: ninety seconds
- Boiled coffee: CGA extraction peaks at two minutes
- Kalita: three minutes, thirty seconds

COFFEE LAB: CGA EXTRACTION DURING BREWING

Generally speaking, the longer a coffee is brewed, the greater the overall extraction from the grounds. In the Coffee Lab, however, we discovered that extraction of chlorogenic acids reaches a maximum after two minutes of brewing with boiling water. This is the longest you need to brew coffee to bring the greatest amount of this healthy phenol into your cup.

EXTRACTION AND TIME

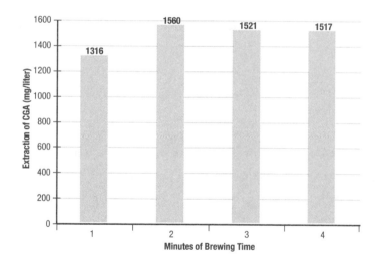

The extraction of CGA increased as brew time increased. After two minutes of boiling, maximum extraction was reached. There was not additional extraction by boiling longer.

2. TEMPERATURE: Raising water temperature speeds chemical reactions and increases extraction. The best coffee roasters run tests on each batch of beans to learn which brew temperature best suits it. In the Coffee Lab we tested brew temperatures from 170 degrees to 212 degrees, and found that water heated to 205 degrees achieves maximum coffee extraction without a burnt taste. (Automatic pour-over devices like Keurig and electric drip machines won't let you set the temperature, of course, but with an electric kettle such as the Bonavita, you can set the temperature digitally before performing a manual pour-over with a Kalita, Chemex, or other device. In this chapter we'll teach you to use all of these methods.)

Some brew techniques use boiled water, so the coffee they produce tastes slightly bitter, but I like them, and the boiling extracts far more of the anti-inflammatory fats cafestol and kahweol. Cowboy coffee, which is boiled right in the pan over an open fire, is gritty and bitter, but what's a cowboy without grit? I use light-roasted African beans for my occasional cowboy coffee, since the grit gives it lots of body that it may otherwise lack. Greek coffee just briefly touches the boiling point, so any resulting bitterness is balanced by the coffee's natural sugars. (Nonetheless, tradition holds that sugars are also added to offset bitterness.)

3. GRIND: The size and shape of ground coffee particles affect the coffee's strength as well as its phenol extraction.

SCAA GRIND DESCRIPTION

DESCRIPTION	SIZE (MM)	# OF PARTICLES	INCREASE IN PARTS/GM	RATIO INCREASE	AREA (SQ./GM)
Whole Bean	6.0	6	–	–	8
Cracked Bean	3.0	48	42	1	16
Coarse Grind	1.5	384	336	8	32
Regular Grind	1.0	1,296	912	22	48
Drip Grind	0.75	3,072	1,776	42	64
Fine Grind	0.38	24,572	21,500	512	128
Espresso Grind	0.20	491,440	466,868	11,115	240

This is the easiest variable to change. I play around with grind when trying a new coffee, starting with a very fine grind and moving incrementally to a coarse one. Because a very fine grind slows the speed of the water's passage through the coffee, it allows more time for extraction. The water also can surround many more particles, so a very fine grind can create a bitter taste from overextraction and pull more caffeine from the beans. I think the medium-coarse grind produces a lovely cup of coffee, and still delivers phenols. As you develop a relationship with a roaster, ask him or her to recommend the temperature and grind best suited to the beans you purchase.

COFFEE LAB: MAXIMIZING PHENOL EXTRACTION WITH GRIND SIZE

Unquestionably, our lab testing showed that the finest grinds extract the most phenols. A very fine grind allows for 50 percent more phenol extraction than a medium grind. Even a medium-fine grind suffers a 30 percent drop in phenols. The high level of extraction in the super-fine grind is the primary reason Greek coffee delivers such noteworthy health benefits.

GRIND SIZE AND EXTRACTION

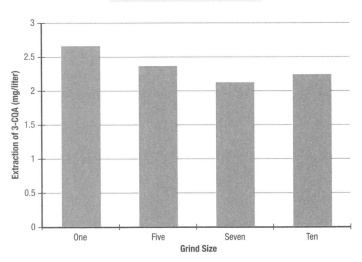

The very finest grind size, "one," yielded the increased greatest extraction of polyphenols. Extraction decreased as grind size. "One" would be a Turkish grind. "Ten" would be a medium-coarse grind. Be sure to match taste with extraction—too fine may be too bitter.

4. WATER-TO-COFFEE RATIO: This ratio determines the strength of the coffee rather than the percent of solubles extracted, and it is absolutely critical to making good coffee. Beethoven was so meticulous about this ratio that each morning he counted precisely sixty beans with which to make his cup of coffee. The SCAA cupping standard puts the ideal ratio at 8.25 grams of whole bean to 150 milliliters or 5.07 ounces of water. That works out to a ratio of 1.63 grams of whole bean to 1 ounce of water. For each brewing technique introduced in this chapter, we'll offer a cheat sheet that tells you the ideal amounts of coffee and water to use.

DR. BOB'S EQUIPMENT LIST

I admit, I'm a coffee geek. I'm sure if you took one look at my kitchen, you'd agree. On my counter resides an industrial-style Mahlkönig EK 43 grinder, the king of grinders, capable of transforming the hardest, light-roasted beans into a fine powder. A highly accurate gram scale measures every milligram of coffee and water that passes through the place. I have devices for preparing coffee a multitude of ways, from a simple saucepan for cowboy coffee to the more sophisticated Elan,[1] Chemex, Kalita, AeroPress, Le Cafetiere, French press, and Turkish ibrik. Then there's the coffee. Bags of freshly roasted coffees from around the globe, including the finest Brazilian Bobolink, Kenyan Gathugu, SL 28, Mexican Chiapas, and Ethiopian Hambela. It's my coffee equivalent to a wine cellar (although the beans don't improve with age!). I use a VST refractometer to measure concentration and extraction yield. Yet even that is not enough; I send my coffees to the chemistry lab to be tested for health benefits!

Coffee paraphernalia doesn't have to overrun your kitchen as it has mine, but you will want to invest in some staples. We've been over what sort of coffee to buy; now we'll look at the other essentials.

SCAA-CERTIFIED BREW DEVICES

Always aiming to encourage high-quality brewing, the Specialty Coffee Association of America tests brewing devices and issues certification to those that pass muster. At publication time, SCAA-certified home brewers included the following (visit scaa.org for the most current list):

- Technivorm Moccamaster
- Brazen Plus Customizable Temperature Control Brew System
- KitchenAid Coffee Maker KCM0802
- KitchenAid Pour Over Coffee Brewer (model KCM08010B)
- Bonavita Coffee Maker (model BV1900TS)
- Bonavita BV1900TD 8-Cup Digital Coffee Brewer
- OXO On 9-Cup Coffee Maker
- OXO On 12-Cup Coffee Maker
- Wilfa Precision Coffee Maker
- BUNN 10-Cup Programmable Coffeemaker
- Behmor Brazen Connected 8-Cup Coffee Maker

GRINDERS

Conical burr grinders are better than metal blade grinders because they create more precise, uniform particles, which make better-tasting coffee. Metal blades can shred a bean into a mix of jagged chunks and dusty powder. In the Coffee Lab we found that particles ground by a metal blade ranged in size from 100 to 1,000 micrometers. Those ground by a conical burr grinder measured between 250 and 350 micrometers, and bore a slivered shape that allows better extraction and, ultimately, better taste.

MAHLKÖNIG EK 43: This enormous beast drills through even the hardest beans. Mahlkönig also makes less expensive models ideally suited for home use.

CUISINART: This programmable home grinder has conical burrs and a range of grind settings, and costs less than $100. I've used this in my kitchen and, while fairly expensive, it's very durable.

TURKISH COFFEE HAND GRINDER: Greek coffee requires a powdery, fine grind best achieved with a hand grinder. I take one with me when I travel so I can grind beans in my hotel room. It's tough work, but I love the expression baristas use for hand grinding: "Earn your buzz!" Porlex offers a good one, called the JP-30 Stainless Steel Coffee Grinder, which sells on Amazon for about $55.

BLADE GRINDERS: Use one of these only as a last resort. They'll mash and slice the spectacular beans you've bought, ruining their potential before the water even touches them.

SCALE

I like the Jennings CJ4000 scale, which is very accurate and runs about $25. You can place a carafe on it and zero the scale, then pour in the precise number of grams of water needed for your brew technique.

KETTLE

I recommend the Bonavita 1.0L Variable Temperature Gooseneck Electric Kettle, which allows you to set the precise temperature of the water you'll use to brew your coffee. Boiling water on the stove leads to overextraction and bitter-tasting coffee.

WATER

It may seem picky to make a big deal about the kind of water that you use, but it comprises 98 percent of your coffee, and has enormous influence on its flavor. Rarely is water just water. Read on to learn how its contents affect your coffee, and discover the ideal characteristics of water for brewing a perfect cup. If you don't already, consider filtering your water!

NOT JUST H_2O

A few decades ago a New Yorker opened a pizza shop in Los Angeles. Despite following his original recipe, he found the pizza was no good; the crust didn't have that New York–style texture. This is where David Beeman comes in, a native Californian who once planned to be a chef but, along the way, became so intrigued with the possibilities in water treatment that his life changed course. By altering the mineral content of the Los Angeles water used in the pizza dough, Beeman duplicated New York City water, and, voilà, the pizza was perfect. The store was a success and Beeman duplicated NYC water at each location of what soon became a local chain. Beeman was making it possible to maintain product consistency by developing specific formulas for water and creating treatment systems to adjust the components of water to those specifications.

I learned about Beeman when I was developing our test coffees. He'd begun experimenting with different water characteristics for coffee, and developed a formula for coffee water at Wolfgang Puck's famous Spago restaurant, around the time Starbucks was just getting started. Following the success of their first store in Seattle, Starbucks opened a location in Santa Monica, but the coffee just didn't taste the same. Beeman arrived on the scene. He went to the café at five in the morning to set up equipment to brew the coffee, he tells me. He did a cupping with the shop's filtration system. Then he hooked up his filtration system and duplicated the Seattle water. When the Starbucks representative tasted the first cupping, "He spat it out on the counter," Beeman recalls. "He tasted the second. 'That's my coffee,' he said. 'How do I get it?'"

Beeman became the guru of formulating water for coffee. He established water filtration systems for most of the specialty coffee companies you know. He helped write the SCAA's water quality handbook and create their table of ideal water characteristics for coffee, shown on page 156. "With the right water quality, you can extract completely different flavor profiles from coffee," Beeman says. Before the development of industry-wide standards, water was causing all kinds of trouble. Shipped all over the world, from Costa Rica to Amsterdam and beyond, coffees tasted drastically different in one place than in another. "There got to be this thing where the buyers thought they were being lied to, growers thought the buyers were lying so that they could drop the prices; nobody knew what was going on," Beeman says.

People often ask him if the right water can make cheap coffee taste better. Cheap coffee tastes like cheap coffee, he says. Growers are achieving bean quality phenomenally better than they could years ago, however, so coffee costs are rising significantly. ("It's great for the farmers, because, boy, they need it desperately," Beeman says.) For consumers spending more for better beans, he warns, "With the wrong water, you can make a very expensive coffee taste horrible."

In the table on page 156 you can see that the ideal amount of total dissolved solids (tds) is 150 milligrams per liter. Water with just the right type and amount of minerals works better for coffee than distilled water "because the minerals find a mate in the chemistry of the coffee itself, and will bond to that mate," Beeman says. By contrast, low-mineral water, such as distilled or reverse-osmosis water, will overextract coffee, giving it an ugly astringent taste. If you prepare coffee at home, compare the ideal characteristics to water tests in your locality if you use tap water, or to the labels on spring water. If you're stuck with tap water that doesn't meet specifications, you can remove unwanted elements with a water filter, or by adding a charcoal filter to a Keurig, if you have one, and filtering the water through it. Beeman's company, GC Water, also sells a kit for home use. Most important, your water should have no chlorine, which lends an unpleasant taste. Hard water containing too much magnesium and calcium will take a toll on your equipment and give you a weaker cup.

SCAA IDEAL WATER CHARACTERISTICS

CHARACTERISTIC	
Calcium	30–80 mg/liter
Chlorine	0
Sodium	10 mg/liter
pH	7.0
Alkalinity	40 mg/liter
TDS 3	100–200 (150 mg/liter ideal)
Odor	Clean, fresh, no odor
Color	Clear
Iron	0

BREW TECHNIQUES

The many methods of coffee brewing fall into two categories, known as pour-over and immersion. Pour-overs, as the name connotes, pour a stream of water over a bed of grounds, and coffee drains through a filter to a container below, while immersion techniques allow water to completely envelop the coffee. Pour-overs require a bit more art than immersion techniques since the water must be poured evenly in concentric circles over the grounds. Grind size determines flow rate, so the choice of grind is important. Timing each pour can be critical, too. In short, mastering pour-overs requires practice if you don't use automated devices, such as Keurig or electric drip coffeemakers.

In compiling instructions for the many brew techniques that follow, we found the folks at Barrington Coffee Roasting Company, SCAA, the George Howell Coffee website, and lessons learned from countless test brews to be most helpful. We encourage you, too, to search techniques online, ask your local roaster for tips, and practice to perfect a method you love.

COFFEE LAB: BEST EXTRACTION TECHNIQUES

We're going to teach you to use many brew techniques in both pour-over and immersion categories, but in the following chart we offer a sneak peek at the methods that proved best in the Coffee Lab at extracting phenols.

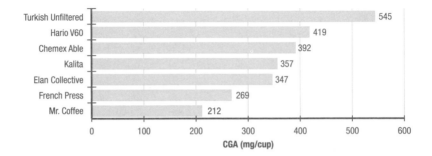

The Coffee Lab tested extraction for popular brewing techniques. The unfiltered Turkish technique yielded the very highest extraction. The Hario, Chemex, Kalita, and Elan all yielded great-tasting cups of coffee. French press yielded a lower extraction due to its larger grind size. Mr. Coffee did well, but its lower temperature yielded a lower extraction.

POUR-OVER

KALITA

This is a favorite pour-over technique for finely ground beans, because the water will still pass through them. (Chemex is similar, but its conical filter retains more water, so with a fine grind, very little coffee passes through its pointed tip.) The Kalita employs an ingenious system with a flatter bottom and three holes to let coffee pass. The Kalita ultrathin filter traps undesirable fats, while allowing more water to pass through than thicker filters do. Getting the proportions exactly right is key to success with a Kalita, so use a gram scale to weigh your coffee and water.

---

1. Measure 28 grams of whole coffee beans on a scale and grind on a medium or fine setting.
2. Fill kettle with water and set to 200 degrees.
3. Place the Kalita Wave Dripper 185 on top of a coffee cup that closely fits the dripper, or on a dedicated Kalita carafe.
4. Place a Kalita 185 filter in the dripper.
5. Spread the coffee grounds evenly in the filter.
6. Place the entire setup (coffee cup or carafe, dripper, and filter) on the scale, and reset the scale to 0.
7. Using a stopwatch or smartphone, pour the 200-degree water into the filter, in concentric circles at timed intervals. Begin the pour at the center of the filter and move outward with your circles, wetting any dry spots. Try to adhere to the following timetable, pouring about 65 grams of water in 15-second intervals, and pausing for 15 seconds between intervals:
   - 0–15 seconds, 65 grams of water poured
   - pause 15 seconds
   - 30–45 seconds, 130 grams of water poured
   - pause 15 seconds

- 1:00–1:15, 195 grams of water poured
- pause 15 seconds
- 1:30–1:45, 260 grams of water poured
- pause 15 seconds
- 2:00–2:15, 325 grams of water poured
- pause 15 seconds
- 2:30–2:45, 390 grams of water poured

8. Coffee should complete draining into the cup or carafe when the stopwatch reaches 3 minutes, 30 seconds. Carefully remove the filter over a wastebasket to dispose, and enjoy your coffee!

TIPS

- If you love this technique but don't have patience in the morning to do the elaborate pour, try this abbreviated method: Pour water over the coffee grounds slowly until all have been wetted. Pause to allow the coffee to bloom. Good coffee will rise and bubbles will form. Then, slowly pour the rest of the water over the grounds. Once the majority of the coffee has passed through the filter, enjoy!

- If you want to make a half cup, use the Kalita 155 filter, and cut the amounts of coffee and water by half, to 14 grams and 195 milliliters.

BOB ARNOT, M.D.

- Store your filters in a cup so they retain their shape and don't sag.

CHEAT SHEET
- Water: 390 grams
- Coffee: 25–29 grams
- Grind: medium
- Temperature: 200–205 degrees
- Time: 3 minutes, 30 seconds

CHEMEX

Chemex is the most popular pour-over device in the United States, according to the National Coffee Association. It offers a grand and luxurious way to make coffee, and I love the equipment, from the elegant pitcher to the glass kettle, and the sophisticated filter system that sops up fats, preventing them from dripping into your coffee. The only pour-over with enough users to be listed in national usage data, Chemex was the official pour-over of the White House in 2016.

INSTRUCTIONS

1. Measure 25–29 grams of whole coffee beans on a scale and grind on a medium-coarse setting.
2. Fill kettle and set to 200 degrees.
3. Heat the carafe by rinsing it with hot water. Wet the filter and place it in the intake funnel of the carafe.
4. Spread the coffee grounds evenly in the filter.
5. Place the Chemex on the scale and reset it to 0.
6. Using a stopwatch or smartphone, pour the 200-degree water into the filter, in concentric circles at timed intervals. Begin the pour at the center of the filter and move outward with your circles, wetting any dry spots. Try to adhere to the following timetable, pouring 130 grams of water in 20-second intervals, and pausing for 40 seconds between intervals:
   - 0–20 seconds, 130 grams of water poured
   - pause 40 seconds
   - 1:00–1:20, 260 grams of water poured
   - pause 40 seconds
   - 2:00–2:20, 390 grams of water poured
7. Coffee should complete draining into the carafe by 3:30–4 minutes. Carefully remove the filter over a wastebasket to dispose, and pour the coffee into a porcelain mug. Enjoy!

- If you're in a hurry, you can pour water onto the grounds until you have a bloom, wait 45 seconds, then slowly pour over the rest of the water. This isn't the official technique, but still produces a good cup of coffee.

CHEAT SHEET

- Water: 390 grams
- Coffee: 25–29 grams
- Grind: medium coarse
- Temperature: 195–205 degrees
- Time: 4 minutes

FINE-TUNING KALITA AND CHEMEX

- If your coffee tastes weak or sour, it may be underextracted. Correct by adjusting the grinder two stops finer.
- If your coffee tastes bitter or too strong, it may be overextracted. Correct by adjusting the grinder two stops coarser. Overly hot water can also cause bitterness; reduce temperature setting by 5 degrees.

THE ELAN COLLECTIVE

The Elan Collective Pour-Over Brewer is the best pour-over device I've found for very fine grinds, which deliver the highest extraction of phenols. Most other techniques, even Chemex, choke with very fine grinds, meaning that the grinds sop up the water so that very little coffee trickles out of the filter. The Elan brewer, like the other tools in the Collective, was designed by two friends with a shared passion for coffee, barware, and simplistic style. The device has no filter, but is made of a wire mesh of just the right size to allow water to pass easily through extrafine grinds, within three minutes. For those of you who want the added anti-inflammatory benefit of the fats cafestol and kahweol, this device will let through up to one hundred times more of them than filters do. Beware that too much fat in your coffee can raise your cholesterol, so this technique is good for a couple of cups a day. Enjoy!

INSTRUCTIONS

1. Measure 28 grams of whole coffee beans on a scale and grind on the finest setting available on an electric grinder, or use a Turkish hand grinder.
2. Fill kettle and set to 212 degrees.
3. Spread the coffee grounds evenly in the Elan.
4. Place the brewer on top of a coffee cup on the scale and reset it to 0.
5. Using a stopwatch or smartphone, pour the 212-degree

water into the filter, in concentric circles at timed intervals.

6. Begin the pour at the center of the filter and move outward with your circles, wetting any dry spots. Pour 65 grams of water in 15-second intervals, pausing for 15 seconds between intervals. After the first 65 grams, stir gently with a fork. Wait for the water to settle, then continue pouring gently in concentric circles, adding 65 grams every 30 seconds until you have reached the total 340 grams.

7. Once all the water has been poured onto the grounds, gently stir with a fork to break up any clumps of dry coffee. Be very careful not to upset the brewer and spill the coffee.

8. Coffee should complete draining into the mug by 3 minutes. Lift the Elan off the mug, empty grounds into a wastebasket, and enjoy!

CHEAT SHEET

- Water: 340 grams
- Coffee: 28 grams
- Grind: extrafine
- Temperature: 212 degrees
- Time: 3 minutes

- If the coffee is too bitter for your taste, you can back off of the grind to a slightly coarser grind. In our Coffee Lab tests, we found that stirring the coffee as you brew it (as described earlier) achieves much higher extraction. (Be careful not to spill, as the brewer sits on top of your cup.) Our measurements detected at least 305 more polyphenols in cups of coffee brewed with this technique.

HARIO V60-02

The Hario V60-02 coffee dripper is another excellent pour-over technique for very fine grinds, which enables you to get that higher level of phenol extraction. With the V60, you'll find that water passes through even the finest Turkish grinds in just a few minutes. Keep in mind that this is the healthiest of grinds, but may be bitter in taste. You can learn to savor a slightly bitter taste laced with enormous benefits, or try a coarser grind.

INSTRUCTIONS

1. Measure 28 grams of whole coffee beans on a scale and grind on the finest setting available on an electric grinder, or use a Turkish hand grinder.

2. Fill kettle and set to 205 degrees.

3. Wet the filter and place it in the intake funnel of the V60.

4. Spread the coffee grounds evenly in the filter.

5. Place the V60 on the scale on top of a coffee cup and reset it to 0.

6. Using a stopwatch or smartphone, pour the 205-degree water into the filter, in concentric circles at timed intervals. Begin the pour at the center of the filter and move outward with your circles, wetting any dry spots. Pour 65 grams of water in 15-second intervals, pausing for 15 seconds between intervals. Wait for the water to settle, then continuing pouring gently in concentric circles, adding 65 grams every 30 seconds until you have reached the total 340 grams.

7. Coffee should complete draining into the cup by 3 minutes. Carefully remove the filter over a wastebasket to dispose, and enjoy!

TIPS

▪ If you're in a hurry, you can pour water onto the grounds until you have a bloom, wait 45 seconds, then slowly pour over the rest of the water. This isn't the official technique, but still produces a good cup of coffee.

▪ Fine-tuning: Correct for bitterness by adjusting the grind two stops coarser.

CHEAT SHEET

- Water: 340 grams
- Coffee: 28 grams
- Grind: extrafine
- Temperature: 205 degrees
- Time: 3 minutes

KEURIG

Pod devices account for 29 percent of the home coffee market. The Keurig machine, which has the largest market share, is an ingenious piece of engineering that is able to complete a pour-over extraction cycle with minimal mess and time. I've gone over the engineering and it's really amazing how much thought went into this device. Its pros are ease of use and individual customization, so that everyone in the household can have what they want. My four-year-old can prepare a decent cup of coffee with a Keurig!

1. He lifts the lid.
2. He puts in the cup.
3. He lowers the lid.
4. He presses the button for the size cup he wants.

Coffee aficionados turn their noses up at pod devices. Here are a few reasons why. Compared to a manual pour-over, the cups contain far less coffee with less surface area exposed. While most pour-over systems use 25 to 28 grams of coffee, traditional K-cups contain as little as 9 grams, and the extraction time is too short. This results in low extraction of polyphenols. Traditional K-cups aren't recyclable, although improvements are planned. The coffee within them may not be the quality you can buy from a great roaster. And . . . the beans are preground.

In 2016, Keurig submitted new, special reserve K-cups to Coffee Review and earned some excellent scores, using more coffee and terrific beans, such as their Organic Ethiopian Yirgacheffe, which scored a 91.

We made a K-cup when researching this book to see if it was possible to get high extractions of CGAs with the device. We asked Intelligent Blends to make cups with eleven and fourteen grams of coffee respectively, combining a finer grind with a coarser one. The extraction was dramatically better, with 13,527 milligrams per kilogram of the CGA known as 3-CQA, compared to a dark-roast K-cup that had 1,968 milligrams per kilogram of 3-CQA, and a light roast that held 8,135 milligrams per kilogram.

TIPS

- Buy K-cups that have more coffee; some pods contain fourteen grams.
- Intelligent Blends sells biodegradable K-cups in three grind sizes, from fine to coarse. The fine grinds enable better extraction, while the coarser ones allow water to pass through quickly.
- Buy better, whole bean coffee, grind it fresh, and load into a reusable K-cup. I have developed one of these, which holds about fourteen grams of coffee. Ekobrew also makes one, which holds a whopping twenty grams of coffee! With reusable cups, whole families can use a single device to make fast, fresh coffee, even if they love grinding their own artisanal beans.

---

1. Grind 14 or 20 grams of beans on a medium-to-fine setting and add to a reusable K-cup.
2. Place the cup in the Keurig brewer and close the lid.
3. Press the button for the largest cup. If you get too little coffee in the cup, you have used too fine a grind.

ELECTRIC DRIP (BONAVITA, MR. COFFEE, CUISINART, KITCHENAID, ETC.)

Like Keurigs, electric drip machines such as Mr. Coffee and others like it get snubbed by true coffee aficionados; however, these devices dominate the market in American kitchens. In addition to being delightfully inexpensive, the machines proved shockingly good at extracting phenols. The large bed for the coffee grounds allows for an even extraction that helped the Mr. Coffee we tested rank above Chemex and just below Kalita in delivering phenols. Because it's the only electric drip machine that is SCAA certified, we've provided instructions here for using the Bonavita coffee brewer. Follow the instructions included with the device for corresponding weights of coffee and water.

1. Fill the reservoir to the desired water line.
2. Weigh coffee to desired strength and grind on a medium setting.
3. Place the filter in the cone, rinse with water, and fill with coffee.
4. Spread the grounds evenly in the filter.
5. Place the cone atop the carafe, and set inside the brewer.
6. Turn brewer on.
7. When brew cycle is complete, remove the cone, discard grinds, and pour.

TIP

- Brew times will vary depending on the number of cups brewed. Shorter brew times (fewer cups) can take a slightly finer grind.

A NOTE ON ESPRESSO

We've examined how increased temperature, decreased grind size, and increased time all increase the extraction of polyphenols. There is a fourth variable: pressure. Espresso rapidly extracts coffee grinds with very high pressure.

Neither a pour-over nor an immersion technique, espresso is known as an infusion technique, made with very fine grinds and boiling water. Espresso has a fascinating history. Rumor has it that factory owners in Italy in the early 1900s wanted their workers back quickly from breaks, and couldn't wait three minutes or more for pour-over coffees to be prepared. Espresso was fast, completed in just forty-five seconds. The cup was small, so workers received their coffee and drank it quickly to keep captains of industry happy. Now a hint of luxury elevates espresso because it's made to order for individual customers.[2]

Many espresso blends contain beans with darker roasts, but this needn't be. You can use a lighter roast in espresso and still get a great cup of coffee. Combining high-quality beans, lighter roasts, high water temperature, and ultra-fine grind size, espresso can produce a superb extraction. One study showed 188 milligrams of phenols in just a small cup of espresso. Pretty impressive!

When ordering espresso, just ask the barista for a light-roasted high-quality bean instead of the usual espresso beans. I love Kenyan coffees or Colombian Huila for espresso.

IMMERSION

Immersion techniques allow water to completely envelop the coffee grounds for fuller and more even extraction. They are among the easiest and least expensive ways to brew coffee. An AeroPress costs a mere $29, cowboy coffee is made in a simple saucepan, and even an ibrik used to make Turkish coffee costs just $69. Most of these techniques are also highly portable and therefore great for the office or travel.

AEROPRESS

Manual pour-over techniques require such precision that the quality of the coffee varies substantially depending on the experience of the pourer. Honestly, I'm pretty hit-or-miss with some of them, and I like the AeroPress because it is much easier to get right. We recommend a medium grind for the best coffee. You can use a fine grind with full immersion techniques to get optimal extraction of phenols, but be very careful putting fine grinds in the AeroPress; the added pressure required to depress the plunger can end up blowing the coffee and grinds out of the device, making a real mess! As with other brewing techniques, several methods have been developed for using an AeroPress. The following is a method that I learned from my local roaster.

1. Measure 14 grams of whole coffee beans on a scale and grind on a medium setting. (For stronger coffee, grind 20–22 grams.)

2. Fill kettle with 235 grams or 200 ml of water and set to 205 degrees. (Alternatively, bring water to boil on the stove, remove, and let cool for 30 seconds.)

3. Position the AeroPress plunger upside down so the rubber end faces the ceiling. Invert the brewing chamber and carefully place it onto the plunger, stopping when the plunger extends about a half inch into the chamber.

4. Using the AeroPress funnel, pour the ground coffee into the chamber.

5. Using a stopwatch or smartphone, spend 25 seconds pouring the water into the chamber.

6. Wait 10 seconds.

7. At 35 seconds, stir the slurry with a spoon so that all the coffee grounds are exposed to water.

8. Place the paper filter in the cap, and screw the cap onto the brewing chamber.

9. Holding the AeroPress where the plunger and chamber meet, turn the device over and place it onto a mug. (Confirm before brewing that the AeroPress fits the mug.)

10. For 1 minute, slowly press the plunger into the brewing chamber. Stop as soon as air hisses from the chamber, when the plunger is about a half inch above the filter.

11. Enjoy fresh brewed coffee as is, or add more water to dilute if desired.

12. To dispose of the grounds, hold the AeroPress over a trash can, filter down. Unscrew and remove the cap. Press the plunger all the way down to eject the grounds.

TIP

- AeroPress makes both paper and metal filters. Either is fine, but know that the metal filters (which come in medium- and fine-grind sizes) allow more cafestol to pass into your cup. Cafestol, which we discussed in chapter 1, is a highly anti-inflammatory fat that may play a role in fighting diabetes. Too much of it, however, can raise cholesterol. The pressure used to push water through the AeroPress filter may send more cafestol into your coffee than you'll get when using Chemex and Kalita.

CHEAT SHEET

- Water: 235 grams
- Coffee: 14 or 20–22 grams
- Grind: medium
- Temperature: 195–205 degrees
- Time: 2 minutes

FRENCH PRESS

The French press scored the lowest of all the techniques we tested in the Coffee Lab for extracting chlorogenic acids. This technique also allows unwanted fats and even some grounds to pass into your coffee, making it the least effective at extracting health benefits. It is an elegant device that's easy to use, so if you like it, just be sure to use a coarse grind. You can easily remove some of the fats and grounds by pouring your coffee through a filter into your cup.

INSTRUCTIONS

1. Heat the carafe by rinsing it with hot water.
2. Measure 40 grams of whole coffee beans on a scale and grind on a coarse setting.
3. Bring 400 grams of water to boil.

4. Place the press on your scale and add ground coffee.

5. Gently shake the press to even out the coffee bed, replace on scale, and set to 0.

6. Pour 80 grams of boiling water onto the grounds. Stir coffee and water with a wooden spoon.

7. Wait 30 seconds.

8. Pour in the remaining water and let steep for 4 minutes.

9. Remove the press from the scale and place on the counter or other hard, stable surface.

10. Slowly press the plunger firmly to the bottom. Pour and enjoy!

TIP

- Blue Bottle Coffee Company advises using fifteen to twenty pounds of pressure when depressing the French press, and suggests practicing this on a bathroom scale to get the feel of it (https://bluebottlecoffee.com/preparation-guides/french-press).

CHEAT SHEET

- Water: 400 grams
- Coffee: 40 grams
- Grind: coarse
- Temperature: boiling
- Time: 4 minutes

COWBOY COFFEE

Two aspects of boiled coffee make it excellent at extracting chlorogenic acids and other phenols: the fiercely hot temperature and the physical agitation of boiling water. In the Coffee Lab, we determined that extraction of beneficial phenols peaks after two minutes of boiling. Now you have a very healthy brew; the downside is that boiling overextracts coffee, bringing out undesirable elements that taint the way it tastes. But, if you're a cowboy struggling to rouse yourself after spending a cold night on the ground, you probably won't care!

The era of the American cowboy began in the 1880s, with mounted men driving vast herds across the grueling landscapes of the West. You've got to be tough as nails to drink the coffee they drank—yet there are people who love it. Gone are the sophisticated tastes of the pour-over, replaced by some bitterness and raw grit in the cup. The health benefits are staggering, though, and they come easy and cheap. You need only a hand grinder, a saucepan, and a hot fire.

Whether you're a cowboy or a camper, if you've spent the night on the cold, hard ground, any hot cup of caffeine is going to taste great. There are no fussy rules for making cowboy coffee, but we'll give you basic instructions for fixing it on the trail, as well as a slightly refined method for use in the kitchen.

INSTRUCTIONS FOR COWBOY COFFEE ON THE TRAIL

1. Pour 8 ounces of water into a tin saucepan.
2. Grind 2 tablespoons of coffee with a Turkish hand grinder. If you're really tough, double up on the coffee to make a cup of "six-shooter," coffee that can stand up on its own!
3. Bring water to boil over a fire.
4. Toss the finely ground coffee into the water and stir.
5. Wait 4 minutes, or at least 2 if you're impatient.
6. Set your pot on the ground to cool for a minute or two and let the grounds settle to the bottom.
7. Slowly pour coffee into a tin cup, leaving most grounds in the bottom of the pot.
8. Drink your coffee, grit and all!

BOB ARNOT, M.D.

INSTRUCTIONS FOR COWBOY COFFEE AT HOME ON THE RANGE

1. Measure 22.5 grams of coffee on a scale and grind on an ultrafine setting.
2. Fill Bonavita kettle with 300 milliliters of water and set to 212 degrees.
3. Remove the kettle lid and pour the coffee into the boiling water.
4. Wait 4 minutes.
5. Carefully pour the coffee into a cup, stopping before the sludge begins to pour out.
6. Grimace as you swallow. You'll look like a real cowpoke and it will take some of the bite out of the coffee!

TIP

- In our experience, high-altitude coffee beans are best for boiled brews because they generally have high levels of CGA and fruity and floral notes, but often are accused of lacking body. The boiled extraction adds body to the coffee, ideally rounding it out. Since cowboys would be booed out of the corral for drinking an Ethiopian Yirgacheffe, I also recommend the Colombian Popayan Supremo or Colombian Huila Excelso.

WHO DRINKS BOILED COFFEE . . . AND HOW'S THEIR CHOLESTEROL?

NORWEGIANS: The Sami people, who live within the Arctic Circle in northern Norway, where it remains incredibly dark and cold for most of the winter, drink A LOT of coffee, from five to nine cups a day. The Sami drink boiled, unfiltered coffee, so the coffee's fats are present in the solution they drink. Researchers have found that the more coffee the Sami drank, the higher their cholesterol levels climbed.[3] This is the chief reason that doctors warn against drinking too much unfiltered coffee.

DUTCH: Administrants of a Dutch study asked 107 young adults with normal cholesterol levels to consume boiled coffee. Subsequently, the researchers observed a 10 percent increase in total blood cholesterol in those who drank the boiled coffee.[4]

GREEK: Ikarians drinking unfiltered coffee, however, reap great health benefits from it. Cafestol, one of the fats in boiled coffee that isn't present in filtered coffee, may have some benefit in limited doses. Volume, evidently, is the important distinction. The Ikarians were drinking three to five cups of boiled coffee a day, compared to the Norwegians' upper limit of nine cups. The bottom line is this: If you drink more than five cups of boiled coffee a day, check your cholesterol and have a chat with your doctor.

GREEK COFFEE

The Athens-based 2013 epidemiological study that inspired me to begin my own coffee quest observed a direct correlation between drinking Greek coffee and improved vascular function. (Greek and Turkish coffee are one and the same, but the Greeks renamed Turkish coffee during a time of political tension with their neighbor in the 1960s.) The powdery fine grind, which gives water maximum access to the coffee particles, and the boiling water temperature, give the Greeks on the Blue Zone island of Ikaria staggering amounts of chlorogenic acids and other phenols. The study didn't specify which coffee varietal is used by the Ikarians, but their nearest plentiful source of coffee is East Africa, which has the highest-scoring coffees in the world. Greek coffee is very inexpensive to make and is highly portable. All you need is a long-handled copper pot called an ibrik, and a Turkish coffee grinder, which makes the fine, powdery grounds. The combined cost of these is less than $100. (I'm also a fan of the Arzum Mirra electric Greek Coffee Maker, which is very easy to use and runs about $80.) The boiling of Greek coffee is so brief that it retains a very pleasant taste, enhanced by the crema, which boils to the top during preparation. Here's how to create your own Ikarian coffee, the secret to Blue Zone wellness and longevity!

---

1. Measure 20 grams of coffee on a scale and grind using a Turkish hand grinder or burr mill set to fine.
2. Pour 240 milliliters of water into an ibrik.
3. Add coffee and stir. If using cinnamon or other spices, add now.
4. Over low heat on your stove, bring the coffee almost to a boil, then quickly remove the ibrik from heat, and wait 20 seconds.
5. Repeat step 4 twice, so that the coffee has come to a near boil 3 times.
6. Slowly pour the coffee into small, espresso-like cups. A nice crema on top indicates quality beans and good preparation. Drink, leaving grounds at the bottom of the cup.

CHEAT SHEET

- Water: 240 milliliters
- Coffee: 20 grams
- Grind: ultrafine powder
- Temperature: boiling
- Time: 4 minutes

BREW BY BEAN

When I first visited Barrington Coffee Roasting Company in Boston, I was intrigued to find that they had tested and recommend different brewing temperatures depending on the origin of the beans. You can see a few of their matchups here:

http://barringtoncoffee.com/tips/home-brewing-guide/

Another coffee outfit from the UK recommends and sells coffees based on brew technique. Visit their site to select your preferred brewing method to find their recommended beans.

http://www.coffeetastingclub.com

COLD BREW

Cold brew is the hottest new extraction technique of the century. Starbucks, Stumptown, Dunkin' Donuts, and a slew of others are jumping into the game. Why? In a word, convenience. Many people love the taste of cold brew, or prefer cold drinks to hot, but convenience has enormous appeal, too. Cold brew means no long wait at a coffee shop. No waiting for water to boil at home. Ready to drink from a bottle, can, or carton, cold brew allows you to enjoy the energy and performance benefits of coffee instantly. And there's no risk of spilling hot coffee all over your lap while you're driving!

WHAT IS COLD BREW?

All of the brewing techniques we've reviewed so far apply very hot water to coffee grounds over a period of several minutes. Cold brews are prepared by steeping coarsely ground coffee in water at room temperature or in the refrigerator for prolonged periods up to twenty-four hours. Time replaces heat to extract caffeine, taste elements, and polyphenols from the grounds. This process extracts different compounds than hot brewing, resulting in a distinctly different taste and sensory profile; generally, cold brews are sweeter, smoother, and less acidic. Not the same as iced coffee, which is brewed hot, then poured over ice, most cold brew techniques produce a concentrate that can be diluted with water or almond or coconut milk, or added to a smoothie.

ADVANTAGES OF COLD BREW

- **LESS BUZZ**: While cold brew concentrate can contain up to 45 percent more caffeine than hot coffee, diluted cold brew typically is less caffeinated than hot brews. (An analysis of caffeine content run by the Swiss Water Decaffeinated Coffee Company found a caffeinated, di-

BOB ARNOT, M.D.

luted cold brew to contain 159 milligrams of caffeine in an eight-ounce cup, while the caffeinated hot brew analyzed contained 178 milligrams.)[5] If you're overcaffeinated, as I often am, this is great news. The key to this advantage lies in the dilution, however. An article about the caffeine analysis, written by Mike Strumpf, Director of Coffee Quality at Swiss Water Decaffeinated Coffee Company, indicates that if you drink concentrate straight, you may get as much as 518 milligrams of caffeine per eight ounces (which far exceeds the recommended daily limit for many Americans). Making cold brew with decaf is also a great option. Even with minimal caffeine, the cold brew still contains less than hot. The Swiss Water decaf cold brew delivers only six milligrams in an eight-ounce cup versus twelve milligrams for a decaf hot brew.

- **REFRESHING:** When it's hot outside, cold brews serve up a refreshing alternative to hot coffee. As an athlete, I use coffee to train, but I don't want to increase my body temperature with hot beverages, so cold brew offers a perfect alternative that's refreshing and easy to take with me to practice and competitions.

- **LOWER ACIDITY:** While our Coffee Lab testing showed that coffee is less acidic than many popular beverages, cold brew is even less acidic than coffee brewed hot. The pH measurements of most coffees are in the five-plus range. (Remember, seven is neutral; lower numbers are more acidic, and higher numbers are more basic.) The record high for a cold brew coffee pH is 6.43, which is very close to completely neutral. Cold brew water temperatures never get high enough to degrade or oxidize the coffee. According to the website of the popular Toddy Cold Brew System, cold-brew coffees are approximately 67 percent less acidic than conventional hot coffees.[6]

- **STAYS FRESH:** Cold brew can stay fresh for up to two weeks, which is a game changer for those who are short on time. Whether you've made or purchased your cold brew, store it in the refrigerator in an airtight container, so you avoid staling and the coffee doesn't pick up the flavors of other things in your fridge.

DELIVERY

We'll teach you to make your own cold brew, but you can buy excellent concentrates and ready-to-drink beverages online and in stores. Cold brews allow roasters to deliver consumers a finished product. When selling beans, once the roaster buys, roasts, and packages them, his job is over. The rest (grind, water temperature, water quality, brew technique, time, etc.) is left to the consumer, with ample potential for things to go wrong.

Ready-to-drink cold brew products are available just

about everywhere these days, from convenience stores to grocery stores, gyms, and coffee shops. You'll find some in cans at room temperature, and others in the dairy section of grocery stores. Almost all of these are already diluted, so read the packaging to find out what's in them, and beware of those that are presweetened. If you're new to cold brew, check out these tips and try it out!

- **DRINK IT BLACK:** Roasters work hard to get just the right varietals and grinds to make these extraordinary coffees. The best way to enjoy cold brew is black, right out of the bottle or carton of those diluted with water, so you enjoy maximum benefits. If it's too concentrated for your taste, just add more water.

- **ADD-INS:** A study in the *Journal of Agriculture and Food Chemistry* reports that the simultaneous consumption of milk and coffee may impair the bioavailability of CGAs.[7] So, if you want to add ingredients other than water, the best nondairy choices are almond milk and coconut milk. Most cold brews are smooth enough, however, that there's no need for milk of any kind, as there is to cut through the bitter taste of some hot coffees, so it can be a no-calorie treat for dieters. For those of you who do want a decadent yet healthy coffee drink, we've partnered with two California chefs to deliver amazing recipes using cold brew as a base. You'll find these in chapter 6.

- **TETRA PAK:** Cold brew products found in grocery and convenience stores are typically sold in glass or plastic bottles, but there's an excellent delivery system called Tetra Pak that is set to boom over the next decade as the container of choice. Made by a food packaging company based in Sweden, and found in the dairy section of stores, these containers are shaped like a tetrahedron and look like a glossy cardboard milk carton, but embody a sophisticated technology to keep their contents fresh and great-tasting.

- **NITRO:** Many coffee bars now serve cold brew carbonated with nitrogen, called a nitro brew. The carbonation brings out fantastic flavors from the beans, and provides an ultrafast way to get coffee at a busy bar. Bartenders love nitros because they require no messy preparation; the bartender just pulls the tap and pours it into a glass like a beer. The hottest product is a nitro cold brew in a can, released by Stumptown in 2015. This stuff is delicious and fun, as a profusion of tiny bubbles cascades from the can.

- **SMOOTHIES:** Cold brew also is becoming part of a new coffee craze in gyms. Because coffee can improve speed, power, and endurance, some gyms now are adding cold brew concentrate to preworkout shakes. Try them. They're fantastic!

COLD BREW AT HOME

Fun to experiment with at home, cold brew methods abound, but all are pretty simple to execute. Begin with high-quality, high-phenol beans that are light roasted, because the coarser grinds and cold water temperature extract about a third less polyphenols than hot brewing methods. I recommend using a traditional Latin American bean like a Colombian Huila, so that you still get good levels of polyphenols in your coffee. First we'll teach you a hot brew/crash cold method that won't compromise phenol counts, then introduce several cold brew systems that are sold on Amazon and at specialty coffee shops. (In chapter 6, "Recipes and Pairings," we'll give you a recipe for making cold brew concentrate without a store-bought system.) Each of the systems introduced here comes with directions for use and there are great tutorial videos online, but we'll give you quick summaries. Have fun preparing cold brews. There are no fixed rules. You could even add fruit extracts to your water so that it imbues the coffee with novel tastes as it steeps overnight.

CRASH COLD

One way to create a high-phenol cold coffee is to brew hot, and crash cool. Traditional iced coffee oxidizes while it slowly cools, resulting in a bitterness that has nothing to do with the quality of the beans. (Restaurants don't often use special reserve coffees to make iced coffee, so even when fresh, they usually have a very bland flavor.) How can you win? Crash cooling.[8] It's dead easy: Brew into a container that's been chilled in your fridge and filled with ice.

INSTRUCTIONS

1. Weigh out 200 grams of large ice cubes and place them in a chilled pitcher or carafe.
2. Place your favorite pour-over device such as a Kalita, Elan, or Hario V60 over the pitcher.
3. Grind 60 grams of coffee on a coarse setting and spread evenly in the filter.
4. Heat 500 grams of water to 205 degrees.
5. Pour over the coffee bed as you usually would.
6. Remove the pour-over device after 3 minutes, 30 seconds, and serve over ice.

TIP

- I don't have an ice maker, so my favorite way to use this technique is to fill my Turkish coffee copper pot with 200 milliliters of water and freeze it overnight. In the morning, I grind and spread coffee into my Kalita or Elan, and pour over 500 milliliters of 205-degree water into the cold copper pot. Easy to execute, this method gives me a cold coffee with a taste profile far superior to conventional iced coffees.

FILTRON

Filtron is a cold brew system that is setting the standard for many roasters. Because it is designed to steep coffee in cold water, the Filtron device should be stored in the refrigerator while the coffee brews, for about sixteen hours.

INSTRUCTIONS

1. Place the stopper in the bottom of the large plastic coffee bowl.
2. Wet the filter and position it securely in the bottom of the bowl.
3. Pour 12 ounces of coarsely ground coffee directly into the bowl.
4. Place the coffee guard over the grounds.
5. Fit the water bowl over the coffee bowl and pour 56 ounces of cold water into it, up to the fill line.
6. Store the system in the refrigerator and wait 16 hours.

7. When the time is up, remove the empty water bowl and carefully hold the coffee bowl over a 1.5-liter decanter. Slowly pull the stopper out and rest the bowl on top of the decanter. Let it drain 30–45 minutes into the decanter.

8. Tightly sealed, the concentrate will keep in the refrigerator for several weeks.

TODDY COLD BREW COFFEE MAKER[9]

A chemical engineering graduate of Cornell University, Todd Simpson developed the Toddy in 1964. Creating balanced and smooth coffee, the Toddy works much like the Filtron, but brews at room temperature to produce the concentrate, to which you can add cold water or milk, or hot water for a warm coffee.

INSTRUCTIONS

1. Insert the stopper in the bottom of the brewing container.

2. Wet the filter and place in the bottom of the container.

3. Pour one cup of water into the container, then add six ounces of coarsely ground coffee.

4. Slowly pour three more cups of water over the grounds in a circular motion.

BOB ARNOT, M.D.

5. Add six more ounces of ground coffee. Wait five minutes, then slowly pour in three more cups of water. (Don't stir, just push the grounds floating on top into the water with a spoon.)
6. Let the coffee steep for 12–24 hours at room temperature.
7. Remove the stopper and let the coffee drain into the decanter.
8. Seal tightly and store in the refrigerator for up to two weeks.

COFFEESOCK

CoffeeSock is an even simpler brewing system using a sock-like bag, much like cheesecloth, suspended in cold water. The sock acts as a filter, separating the grounds from the water, ensuring that the coffee is free of grounds.

INSTRUCTIONS

1. Fit the fabric filter over the mouth of the jar.
2. Pour the grounds into the CoffeeSock.
3. Pour a little water over the grounds and pause to let them bloom.
4. Slowly pour remaining water over the grounds.

5. Gather the top of the fabric filter together and tuck it through the attached ring to close the bag. Securely cap the jar.

6. Let the coffee steep in the refrigerator for 16–20 hours. Remove the sock from the jar, drink, and enjoy!

DR. BOB'S COFFEE ROUTINES

We've thrown a lot of instructions at you. If you've combed through a dozen different ways to brew coffee, you may be wondering just where to start in adjusting your coffee routine toward a better cup. After learning all the techniques, I eventually developed coffee routines that I follow at home and on the road that combine bits of the best methods to suit my schedule.

AT HOME: At night I measure thirty grams of beans and put them in the top of my grinder, then fill my Bonavita electric kettle with water. In the morning, I beeline for the kitchen and press the "on" switch on both the grinder and the Bonavita. Within a few minutes, the water reaches 205 degrees. I pour it slowly over the ground beans I've spread in the Kalita. Then, I wait until the coffee has dripped into my cup. Done! This is not the proper, patient, pour-and-wait Kalita technique, but it makes a great cup of coffee. The total time elapsed is three minutes, and, for all but thirty seconds, I'm free to prepare breakfast for my four-year-old.

ON THE ROAD: I can't stand to be away from my artisanal coffees when I travel. So that I can still awaken with those amazing aromas, I take on the road with me the following gear:

- Coffee beans
- Turkish hand grinder or a small electric grinder
- Kalita Wave Dripper 185
- Kalita 185 filters
- Portable beverage warmer called Instant Immersion Heater to heat water

This is my hotel routine. The same gear and technique also can be used at the office:

- Before bed: Eyeball the bean measurement and put them in the grinder. Place the immersion device in a cup of water.
- In the morning: Plug in the immersion device and grind the beans.
- Place Kalita filter into the Kalita Wave.
- Spread the grounds in the filter.
- Slowly pour boiling water over the grounds.
- Let drip, and drink! This routine takes only two minutes, yet powers me for the day with a high-quality coffee. My alternative is the AeroPress, which requires even less room in packing.

HOW TO DRINK A CUP OF COFFEE

When you've completed a complex chemical engineering process that began with coffee beans planted in a far-off land, you should take time to enjoy the fruit of your labor! Too many of us gulp our coffee, losing the opportunity to savor its fantastic aroma and taste. There's an art to enjoying the flavor compounds in coffee, like that of sipping wine, but with even more flavor complexity and without the hangover!

First, smell the aromas that explode from the beans as you grind them. At the end of the brew, bring up your cup and inhale the aromas to benefit from the antioxidants suspended in them. Now comes the fun part. Like an expert barista, make a loud slurp to lift thousands of tiny coffee droplets into your mouth. Slurping coats the taste buds on the tongue and aerosolizes your coffee so that you can actually smell it as you drink. (Most of the taste experience actually comes from our sense of smell.) Finally, chew on your coffee after you drink it.

When you're tasting coffee, try to take note of the following traits:

- **FRAGRANCE.** You want to smell and enjoy the aromatics before you drink, like the people in coffee commercials, raising mugs and breathing deeply through their noses.
- **ACIDITY.** The most misunderstood aspect of coffee,

acidity gives coffee its zest. Like the effervescence in a bottle of Perrier, the light acid carries a sweet and fruity taste with it across your tongue and gives your cup brilliance. Without acid, your coffee will be dull and flat.

- **FLAVOR.** Remember that flavor is a combination of senses received from the taste buds on your tongue and the aromas wafting into your nasal passages.
- **AFTERTASTE.** A great cup of coffee should have a pleasant aroma that remains in the back of your mouth after you swallow. It should not leave your mouth feeling like a dirty ashtray!
- **BALANCE** is the combination of all of the above components, indicating the overall impression of a coffee.

When you've purchased top-quality beans that are expertly roasted, you're well on your way to delicious coffee that will change your life for the better. If you prepare it at home, extracting the most benefits and best flavor from those beans is up to you. Play around with the different techniques. Try out various grinds, temperatures, and brew times. Ask your roaster for his or her advice. As you experiment, remember that coffee performs best with a specific grounds-to-water ratio, so it's worth taking time to measure your coffee and water. Soon, your morning cup will be so much more than a wake-up crutch!

Finally, when you want to buy a cup of coffee at a café, be a snob! Don't accept anything less than a pour-over for the best extractions and tastes. Even if you don't prepare your own coffee at home, knowing the various extraction techniques will impress the barista and your guests, just as your knowledge of fine wines would at a great restaurant. If you do have to settle for premade coffee, look for brew devices called Fetcos, which prepare an excellent cup. Ask servers if they grind their own beans instead of using preground coffee, since this will make a world of difference.

THE RECAP

1. The finest grinds and boiling water will give you the healthiest coffee pulsing with phenols.
2. If that tastes too bitter to be enjoyable, dial back slightly on the temperature and grind, which will still produce a very healthy brew that tastes heavenly.
3. If you're in it for the benefits, Greek coffee is your winner.
4. Runner-up is the Elan: easy to use, inexpensive, and totally portable.
5. Kalita and Chemex win my votes for best across the board, with benefits intact and out-of-this-world taste.
6. Water quality matters!

Q AND A

Q. WHAT HAPPENS TO PHENOLS AFTER YOU GRIND COFFEE?

A. In our laboratory, we found that polyphenols are extremely stable even if exposed to the air for several weeks. So ground coffee is still a good source of polyphenols, but absent much of the taste and aroma you would get from freshly grinding your beans before brewing.

Q. I'M AT THE OFFICE ALL DAY. IF I BUY ONE NEW BREWING DEVICE TO USE THERE, WHICH ONE DO YOU RECOMMEND?

A. Honestly, the easiest is still the Keurig. There are biodegradable K-cups and devices like Ekobrew that allow you to grind your own beans and still use the Keurig brewer. I grind some coffee in the morning and bring it in with an Ekobrew or "My K-cup" system that allows me to use my own ground coffee. Also, Coffee Review rates highly some Green Mountain coffees, which are available in pods. Under our test brand, Dr. Danger, we make a biodegradable K-cup as well.

The other technique I use at the office is a modified Greek or cowboy coffee using the Arzum Mirra electric Greek Coffee Maker, which can be ordered from Amazon. In essence, it's an electrically heated pot. I grind the coffee at home and bring it with me. Then I just plug in the pot, put in the water and coffee, and boil, with no need to worry about water frothing over the sides and onto the counter or stove. The device requires a European plug adapter, as it arrives in an amazing package straight from Turkey.

Q. COULD MY TAP WATER BE RUINING MY COFFEE? DO YOU RECOMMEND A CERTAIN FILTER SYSTEM?

A. Sure. Water can completely ruin a good cup of coffee. It happens at my house, where we have too much calcium in the water. The SCAA specifies ideal components of water for coffee. If your home water is terrible, a filter system can be fitted beneath your faucet, and pitcher filter systems such as Brita are a good, inexpensive alternative.

Q. I WANT TO BREW MORE THAN ONE CUP OF COFFEE AT A TIME. CAN ANY OF THE MANUAL POUR-OVER DEVICES DO THIS?

A. Yes. Some, such as Chemex, are large enough to make several cups at a time. If you're using single-serve devices like Kalita or Elan, try using two devices simultaneously. Boil enough water for several cups and have two Kalitas or Elans resting on top of two cups, then just pour the water over each. Very neat and fast.

Q. **HOW DO YOU PREPARE COFFEE ON THE ROAD?**

A. To be safe, because you never know what will be in a hotel room, I use an electric pot or coil to heat water. I pregrind coffee and bring it along in a bag, but for longer trips I bring a grinder and a scale.

Q. **MY COFFEE GOES RIGHT THROUGH MY POUR-OVER. AM I GET-TING GOOD EXTRACTION?**

A. No. There's too little contact time. You may have several problems. If your grind is too coarse, then the water flows through it too quickly. Alternatively, the water may be pouring through the sides of your filter if the water level rises above the grounds. Pour in increments, pausing between pours, directly onto the grounds.

PART III

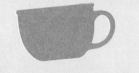

THE COFFEE LOVER'S DIET

CHAPTER 5

THE COFFEE LOVER'S DIET

D o you feel sluggish and unfocused? Do you want to be thinner? More energetic? Do you want to free yourself from sugar cravings? Do you want to be less likely to get sick? If your answers are yes, yes, yes, yes, and yes, you will love the Coffee Lover's Diet! You'll experience a true realignment and win freedom from the bad habits that we all pick up over the years. Most important, you won't be miserable while doing so.

Usually, dieting hurts. Your brain feels like someone pulled the power plug. Acid churns in your stomach, searing your insides. Your willpower erodes and you grow weaker with each passing hour. No wonder ordinary dieting has such an astonishingly low success rate. In most diets, reward is the missing element. Reward makes all the difference, and coffee offers a delicious, nearly calorie-free one (just two calories per cup) that you can look forward to all day long. Warm and cozy or cold and refreshing, coffee can give you a sensory experience that's like a minivacation, along with the most potent legal psychic boost around—all while triggering weight-loss mechanisms in your body. This makes coffee an ideal centerpiece for a diet, and one of life's greatest indulgences.

You've read that you can change your life just by changing your coffee: choosing better beans that are light roasted, and leaving out sugar and fattening milk products. Smoky dark roasts pair well with cream and sugar, so it's no surprise that the combination has become the predominant choice of American coffee drinkers, but it robs us of coffee's powerful potential, and burdens us with extra fat. Better beans that are lighter roasted, on the other hand, burst with flavors such as blackberry, raspberry, hazelnut, dark chocolate, cinnamon, and honey. Pairing those flavors with matching foods will make your coffee explode with taste, your antioxidant level surge, and your calorie count plummet.

Drinking coffee in this new way, and taking time to enjoy it, will help you physically and mentally in your efforts to lose weight. Physically, coffee raises metabolism and helps you burn fat, amplifying the effects of your exercise. Mentally, coffee not only rewards you, but also lifts your mood and distracts you from snacking. The tactile ritual of preparing coffee occupies time you may otherwise spend groping for unhealthy snacks. Replacing junky foods and high-sugar, high-fat coffee drinks with premium lean brews will spare you hundreds of calories and loads of fat each day. With the right coffee, an afternoon pick-me-up can deliver renewed energy, focus, and a boost of antioxidants, instead of a sugary high followed by a debilitating blood sugar crash.

While coffee makes this diet unlike any other, fresh, whole foods are its foundation. There are three essential elements: premium coffees, chia/fruit smoothies, and delicious meals made with phenomenal foods. Better coffee beans and generous servings of fruits and vegetables will heal your body with unparalleled levels of antioxidant and anti-inflammatory polyphenols. Filling whole grains, especially chia, will deliver much-needed omega-3 fatty acids, fiber, and calcium. Lean proteins will build your strength and energy without clogging your arteries or padding your waistline.

The Coffee Lover's Diet is a three-phase plan that will teach you to shed unwanted pounds whenever you need to, and then maintain your ideal weight. The meal recipes found in the next chapter are so delicious that I know you'll turn to them again and again, whether dieting or not. You may love most, however, our recipes for specialty coffee drinks that taste utterly decadent, yet contain only pure, nutritious ingredients. It's extremely hard to find healthy alternatives to the indulgent, dessert-like coffee beverages that Americans have come to love, but we have them here. Generally, we recommend drinking premium coffees black, but when you want a treat, or need help weaning off your favorite coffee-shop concoction, turn to these exceptional recipes for hot, frothy toddies and cold blended coffee shakes.

THE COFFEE LOVER'S DIET

Phase I. Initiation: Premium coffees and three smoothies a day

Phase II. Acceleration: Premium coffees, two smoothies, one meal

Phase III. Revival: Premium coffees, one smoothie, two meals

Phase I of the Coffee Lover's Diet, Initiation, is a short-term, fast-acting weight-loss plan that relies on three filling chia/fruit smoothies in place of meals. Flavorful coffees reward you throughout the day with a mood lift, a distraction from snacking, and an energy boost to keep you going. Phase II, Acceleration, replaces one of the smoothies with a solid meal, when you're ready for some extra protein or just need to sink your teeth into something. Phase III marks a true revival. You are slimmer, you feel better, you have more energy. You don't go back to your old habits now; you stick with a smoothie for breakfast and, of course, your coffees, and choose two meals from our bank of recipes for lunch and dinner.

BOB ARNOT, M.D.

This program is totally flexible. We've built it in such a way that you can begin at any phase that fits your needs and lifestyle. Some dieters have spent weeks on Phase I, while others began with Phase II. If you don't think you can drink smoothies until dinnertime, you can begin your diet with Phase III. The Revival phase is a seven-day model based on nutrient-dense, delicious whole foods. It has been carefully analyzed by a nutrition expert and calibrated so that any smoothie, lunch, dinner, and snack combination will amount to roughly 1,500 calories per day. These are foods you can continue to enjoy for the rest of your life, so when you're ready to shift to weight maintenance, you can keep using the model, but eat larger portions. The recipes in the following chapter will tell you how much food to add to reach a two-thousand-calorie-per-day maintenance plan, which is a good benchmark for healthy adults. You'll need to individualize your plan, of course—some lucky people will need more calories, others fewer—and Phase III will introduce a good tool for determining your needs.

In this chapter, we'll look first at how coffee spurs weight loss and enables you to burn more fat every minute that you exercise. We'll introduce you to the power of the chia smoothie. Then we'll walk you through each phase of the Coffee Lover's Diet, and share some success stories along the way. For athletes, we'll offer tips for using coffee to improve your performance in training and in competition.

Next up, you'll find in chapter 6 a trove of original recipes for smoothies, meals, and snacks to make while you're dieting—and when you're maintaining your new shape and higher energy. These delicious recipes, which will take all the guesswork off your plate, were created for us by incredibly talented chefs Mary Barber and Sara Whiteford. Identical twin sisters from Corte Madera, California, Mary and Sara have authored numerous cookbooks and thousands of recipes. They excel at making the healthiest foods taste utterly delicious, in combinations of perfect harmony. If you're hooked on coffee-shop drinks that are loaded with fat and sugar, fear not; Mary and Sara have whipped up a host of phenomenal alternatives for the Coffee Lover's Diet that will be your ticket to freedom. Finally, we'll move on from recipes to pairings, to offer tips for pairing premium black coffees with premium foods for sensory experiences that you can enjoy, guilt-free, for a lifetime.

HOW COFFEE SPURS WEIGHT LOSS

So, it turns out that the world's most popular beverage after water is also the perfect diet food. It just amazes me that we missed this for decades. Look at all that coffee has to offer:

- Sumptuous taste
- Negligible calories

- Zero glucose load, which prevents spikes in blood sugar
- Reduces inflammation
- Burns fat as a fuel during exercise
- Increases metabolic rate
- Improves the body's handling of blood sugar
- Decreases the absorption of fat
- Provides extra energy
- Puts you in a better mood

Caffeine and phenols are the two ingredients in coffee that aid weight loss the most. Let's take a look at what these powerhouses can do.

CAFFEINE INCREASES METABOLIC RATE. If you feel like your engine's running a little faster when you've had a caffeinated beverage, that's because it actually is. Caffeine increases the body's metabolic rate, so it burns more calories, even when you're not exercising. Depending on the amount of caffeine in your coffee, drinking one to three cups may increase your metabolism so that you burn an extra seventy-five to one hundred calories a day.[1] If you replace a caloric snack with coffee, you are creating a terrific calorie deficit. Swap out a four-hundred-calorie doughnut for black coffee, for example, and you are five hundred calories ahead for the day.

COFFEE HELPS YOU PREFERENTIALLY BURN FAT WHILE YOU EXERCISE. This is perhaps the greatest way coffee wrings more from your workouts. Caffeine frees up fatty acids so you can use them as a fuel. This fat-burning mechanism—taking fatty acids right out of your fat stores and burning them immediately—has a profound effect on weight loss, and is the best training improvement I've found in any sports beverage or supplement. Burning free fatty acids instead of sugar allows anyone to *remove fat stores* during exercise. It allows endurance athletes to preserve more muscle fuel stores, enabling them to go faster and farther when racing.

PHENOLS DECREASE THE ABSORPTION OF FATS FROM THE INTESTINE. To best enjoy this effect, look for high-phenol coffees that you can drink with meals so you absorb less fat while digesting. If you eat a high-fat meal, we suggest drinking a medium-roast coffee afterward, because it contains more melanoidin, an important antioxidant that works in the digestive system to decrease the absorption of some fats.

PHENOLS DECREASE THE PRODUCTION OF NEW FAT. An animal study published in 2010 in the *American Journal of Physiology* found that coffee polyphenols (CPP) increased energy expenditure and decreased the production of new fat.[2] The authors noted that "supplementation with CPP significantly reduced body weight gain, abdominal and liver fat accumulation." They concluded that coffee phenols can safely counteract obesity. As our own lab testing showed, many coffees contain few phenols, so buying better beans is crucial to getting these amazing benefits.

BOB ARNOT, M.D.

PHENOLS MAKE FAT LESS DANGEROUS. The phenols in coffee also decrease peroxidation, a process that creates more dangerous fats that can damage cell membranes and contribute to the risk of coronary artery disease.

COFFEE HELPS MAINTAIN WEIGHT LOSS. Keeping weight off is often even harder than losing it. Coffee helps there, too; a study published in 2015 in the *European Journal of Clinical Nutrition*[3] showed that a group of people successful in maintaining weight loss consumed significantly more cups of coffee and caffeinated beverages compared with participants in the general population sample.

COFFEE MAINTAINS MUSCLE MASS. In animal studies of muscle loss due to aging, coffee proved to help maintain muscle mass.[4] Its powerful anti-inflammatory effects, along with a weight-training program, can play an important role in helping you maintain muscle as you age.

PHENOLS IMPROVE EXERCISE PACE. Coffee may be the best exercise aid you'll ever try, because it allows you to work out longer and harder than you otherwise might. CGAs increase your anaerobic threshold during exercise, which allows you to work at a higher pace. Working out at a higher pace means more calories burnt in the same amount of time. The higher the CGA content of your coffee, the more of this effect you reap.

COFFEE IMPROVES SPEED AND POWER DURING EXERCISE. England's University of Birmingham in 2013[5] ran time trial studies with cyclists and triathletes to measure how hard and fast they could go. The results were astonishing. Those who drank coffee beforehand increased their speed by 5 percent, and upped their power from 274 to 292 watts. Those are improvements that most athletes would die for. Anyone can benefit, however, as coffee makes workouts much easier and more pleasant. If you don't work out, you may now be able to tolerate it. You'll feel light and efficient. Your metabolism will be cranking. Since you'll burn more calories every minute you exercise, you'll take off more weight. Even if you simply walk for exercise, you'll find more spring in your step.

USE YOUR NOSE!

Professional Q Graders, known as "cuppers," who test the aroma and taste of coffees, always smell coffee before they sip it. You should, too, as some of the antioxidants brimming in coffee are delivered through its aroma.

COFFEE HELPS PREVENT TYPE 2 DIABETES

Roughly 10 percent of Americans suffer from diabetes.[6] By far the most common, type 2 diabetes causes blood sugars to rise abnormally and prevents the body from using insulin and transporting blood sugar properly, sometimes

BOB ARNOT, M.D.

leading to complications such as nerve damage, eye problems, high blood pressure, kidney disease, heart disease, and stroke. Lifestyle changes like healthy eating and exercise go a long way in controlling this devastating condition. Coffee, too, can play a role in preventing it, through several mechanisms that help clear blood sugar.

A vast study of more than ninety-three thousand people conducted by scientists in Denmark in 2015[7] observed that high coffee intake was associated with low risk of obesity, metabolic syndrome, and type 2 diabetes. Although researchers did not find genetic evidence of the link, they observed that coffee worked to reduce these health risks even in participants who were overweight or had high blood pressure and cholesterol.

As you lose weight, improve your diet, and drink more coffee, you should see an improvement in your fasting blood sugar and in your cholesterol level, as well as in results of inflammation tests such as CRP (C-reactive protein). If you have diabetes, you may find that many indicators of the disease improve.

GET YOUR HEAD IN THE GAME

We've seen how the ingredients in coffee boost weight loss physically, but coffee also eases the mental hurdles in dieting. It delivers delicious, frequent taste rewards, which are critical to any successful diet plan. The act of preparing coffee, especially with manual techniques, is an artful ritual that occupies and distracts when the urge to snack strikes. Chemically, coffee serves up a powerful mood boost. We discussed in chapter 1 the abilities of caffeine and phenols to impact brain chemistry to make us feel happier. Having a good-tasting reward gives us pleasure, but coffee is actually capable of improving mood.

All of these factors make coffee an excellent diet facilitator. An interesting new concept in dieting that's emerged from research in Sweden focuses on dieting barriers and facilitators. Success comes with removing barriers, like poor eating habits, busy schedules, and lack of self-control, and with implementing facilitators, like rewards and easy-to-follow plans. Using coffee to help you lose weight couldn't be easier; all you have to do is increase your consumption and pick coffees with high phenol levels.

The plans that follow aim to bring you frequent rewards and all of the health benefits that come with a high intake of antioxidant, anti-inflammatory phenols. This means a good deal of coffee. However, you don't have to drink three to five cups of caffeinated coffee a day to see benefits, and you shouldn't do so if you're slow to metabolize caffeine. (When we say "cup" we mean about 250 milliliters, or 8 ounces of coffee. For reference, a Starbucks "short" size contains about 240 milliliters; a "tall" contains about 350 milliliters.) Switching to high-phenol coffee and skipping cream and sugar, even if you drink only one cup in the mornings, will give you better-tasting coffee, less fat, fewer calories, and more antioxidants. As a slow caffeine metabolizer myself, I urge you to try the high-phenol decafs recommended in this chapter, and in the Resources section, which are big on taste and benefits. Remember to drink plenty of water as well, at least sixty-four ounces, or eight cups, a day.

POWER OF THE SMOOTHIE

The chia smoothie has been the mainstay of my nutrition for years. Most people love the mouthfeel of a thick, cold, smoothie, but these fun shakes that straddle the line between food and beverage have benefits that go way beyond pleasure. First, by blending foods, you minimize your meal prep time and let the blender do the work. Second, blending your food aids digestion, giving your overworked digestive track a break. And here's the clincher: Blending foods helps you maximize your intake of crucial nutrients. How many of you eat nine servings of fresh fruits and vegetables a day? Not many, I bet. I've never much liked kale or spinach. Blended with fruits and yogurt in a smooth, frosty liquid, however, those superfoods are undetectable, except for their vibrant green hue.

The fruits and vegetables in the smoothies you'll learn to make in this book will give you a windfall of polyphenols that complement those you'll get from your improved coffee routine. Also pivotal to your diet, however, is chia. I wrote a whole book about these incredible seeds. Chia is one of the healthiest foods in the world, an ancient grain whose seeds are spectacular for weight loss. Best absorbed when they are microsliced or ground, these miracle seeds are high in protein and omega-3 fatty acids, with an ultra-low glucose load. They absorb liquid and expand to form a gel in your stomach, which keeps you feeling full for hours. No more hunger while dieting!

The whole grain that fueled the success of the ancient Aztec warriors, chia packs more omega-3s than any whole food—*eight* times more than a piece of salmon. Chia has six times more calcium than milk, three times more iron than spinach, and twice the fiber of bran flakes. Toss a few tablespoons of ground or microsliced chia in a smoothie with kale, blueberries, Greek yogurt, and a few other tasty superfoods, and you have every bit of nutrition you'll need all day, in a delicious, easily made, portable meal. So potent is this shake that it will give you more anti-inflammatory and antioxidant compounds than most Americans consume in a month. It will make you feel the best you ever have!

I aim to have six tablespoons of cold-pressed ground chia a day, mostly in my smoothies. That amount will cause bloating or reflux if chia is new to your digestive system, so it is important to start with one tablespoon and work your way up. You may find your limit to be anywhere from three to six tablespoons per day, spaced throughout the day.

If you like to eat something different every day, you'll love our unique and varied smoothie recipes in chapter 6. One of the secrets to great smoothies is freezing the fruits, and even the greens if you wish, which preserves their farm goodness, and gives your shake a nice, cold thickness without watering it down with ice. (Freezing diminishes the taste of greens if you're not a fan.) Remember that the smoothies are meant to serve as meal replacements; our blended coffee drinks, on the other hand, can serve as decadent, yet nutritious treats. Having found that I do best with a limited list of foods, I stick primarily to the recipe called Dr. Bob's Super Smoothie, which I make almost every morning.

Most of the dieters featured in this book used a brand of chia called E'lan, which is prepared with a sophisticated, cold-press grinder that maximizes the nutrients in chia without destroying the anti-inflammatory compounds and omega-3 fats. Many other quality brands of chia can be found at Whole Foods, health food stores, and online. E'lan can be purchased online at vital2life.net.

Now, I know many of you are thinking, *Well, I travel*, or *I take the bus to work. How can I possibly sip a smoothie all day?* I fill a few thermos bottles with my smoothie in the morning, and take them with me when I'm on the run. They last me until evening, and I'm never hungry because the fiber and protein are so satiating. Truthfully, you will continue to hanker for sugary or fried foods, or whatever is your personal vice, but you won't be hungry, and you won't feel down or light-headed. Here's why:

- The smoothie's **glucose load** is extremely low so that your blood sugar stays steady all day long.
- You're satisfying your body's **micronutrient hunger** for all the minerals and vitamins that may be missing from your diet.
- The combination of **chia and kale** keeps you extremely full. You'll only be able to sip this smoothie through the day; it's not a gulper. Mine lasts until early evening. I don't get reflux or symptoms of overfullness because I just sip it.

- You'll get more anti-inflammatory compounds in a single day than most Americans do in a month, so you'll feel wonderful. You may notice that symptoms of various chronic illnesses ease as your body's inflammation recedes.

SMOOTHIE + COFFEE?

Yes. You drink the smoothie throughout the day, and your intermittent coffee treats complement its fruity flavors. The ideal pairing for these smoothies is a high-altitude East African coffee that enhances the fruit flavors of the smoothie. Ethiopian Hambela is a great choice, especially if you have blueberries in your smoothie.

PHENOMENAL PHENOLS

Of all the foods and beverages we've tested in the lab, coffee has the broadest range of phenols. Some wonderfully beneficial phenols, however, aren't present in coffee, so you'll want to include in your diet certain fruits and vegetables to round out your phenol intake. Sources of phenols that are complementary to those in coffee include:

- Blueberries (wild Alaskan preferred)
- Green tea (ceremonial grade)

- Fresh grapes
- Red wine

Polyphenols are a type of phytochemical, a broader term for nutrients found in plant-based foods. My colleague Dr. David Nieman, of the Human Performance Lab at NCRC, advises us to eat as wide a variety as possible of fruits, vegetables, nuts, seeds, and whole grains to get the highest amount of phytochemicals. Every food has something different to offer, he says.

This is no casual recommendation. A renowned European study conducted over twelve years showed that people with the highest intakes of polyphenols had a 30 percent decreased risk in all causes of death compared to those with the lowest intakes. Very few medications or therapies in medicine lend that degree of benefit!

As impressive as those results are, Dr. Nieman says they may be modest compared to newer studies. While the European study examined phenol content in urine output, newer studies are able to measure the phenol content in what people eat. A study published in *The American Journal of Clinical Nutrition* in 2015 found an even greater protection: The highest intakes of the polyphenols (flavonoids) were associated with 60 percent lower risk of all-cause mortality than the lowest intakes.[8]

Clearly, consuming a broad range of phenols benefits

health and disease resistance. Just as the Ikarians fare incredibly well from the combined effects of their healthy coffee and Mediterranean diet, you'll feel best if you complement your high phenol coffee with colorful fruits and vegetables. A study of phenol intake in various diets shows that in Mediterranean diets, fruits are the second highest source of phenols after coffee. Most Western diets contain less fruit, providing only 13 percent of total phenol intake. (Coffee provides 41 percent, and tea 17.4 percent.)

Fruit smoothies offer an excellent way to increase this percentage. Try to slip in as many phenols as you can, I've suggested blueberries, which often rank highest among fruits for phenols. You may also consider grapes, cherries, plums, apricots, and peaches. High-phenol vegetables include kale, spinach, leeks, and cherry tomatoes. To create a beverage that is super rich in phenols, try adding cold brew coffee to your fruit smoothies. The combination is one of the best measures imaginable to improve your overall health while you lose weight. Our Blueberry Pomegranate Frappe, found among the coffee drink recipes in the next chapter, provides a perfect example.

The chart on page 226 is a great reference for foods and beverages that are highest in polyphenols.

HIGH-PHENOL FOODS

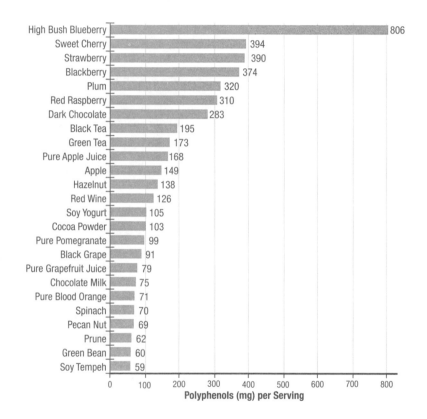

These foods and beverages contain the highest amounts of other phenols important to health. They are different from and highly complementary to the phenols in coffee.

BOB ARNOT, M.D.

PHASE I. INITIATION

I use this plan to get back on track and trim down whenever I've spent weeks traveling and overeating. I broke my pelvis in a ski training run while writing this book, and after my recovery, I used it to get down to my best weight in two decades. Phase I takes discipline, but it always works. The smoothies will keep you full and satisfy all your nutritional needs, and the coffees will keep you happy and energized. The plan couldn't be simpler:

- **CHIA SMOOTHIES: BREAKFAST, LUNCH, AND DINNER**

  Choose my Super Smoothie or one of the smoothie recipes in chapter 6, and make three servings in the morning (or at night for the following day). You may need to multiply the recipes to reach your targeted calorie totals. Sip your smoothies throughout the day. The chia will make you feel overly full if you gulp them down quickly.

- **COFFEES: HIGH-PHENOL COFFEES, IDEALLY BLACK, THROUGHOUT THE DAY**

  Have a cup of coffee when you wake. You'll start burning fat within the hour and feel alive again with a nice, smooth onset of caffeine-induced wakefulness.

  Try not to pack too much caffeine into the first hour or

so after you wake up. Remember, it takes almost an hour to feel the full effects, so you'll overload if you drink too much at once. Two hours is a nice interval after which to have your second cup.

Make a coffee whenever you feel like snacking, or when you want something warm or need an energy boost. Drink one an hour before you work out. You'll love how you feel while exercising!

If you buy coffee from a café, ask for single-origin beans from high-altitude countries near the equator, with the lightest roast offered. Ask for a pour-over. Be aware of varying caffeine content.

Switch to decaf as needed.

Skip the cream and sugar. This is easier than you might think when you're drinking high-quality beans with lighter roasts. Tamas Buday, the three-time Olympic kayaker who traded in his old coffee for light-roasted high-phenol brews, says this of making the switch: "I thought the taste was so good, I stopped drinking my coffee with milk. Now I just drink it pure. I wouldn't even think of putting milk in my coffee. The aroma, the scent, is so delicious it does not need milk."

■ **SNACKS**

Choose a snack from our recipes in chapter 6, once or twice per day, but only if you're hungry.

Exercise in the morning if your schedule allows. With nothing but coffee on board, you'll start burning fat right away.

If you prefer to exercise in the evening, try drinking a coffee an hour beforehand, decaf if you're caffeine sensitive. You can sip your smoothie throughout your workout, if you like. It's a perfect fuel, and reliably staves off hunger.

During the early phases when your calorie intake is restricted, try moderate cardio like walking or cycling, yoga or strength training.

COFFEE SUGGESTIONS BY THE CLOCK

I like to drink specific coffees during different periods of the day to get maximum benefits and a variety of taste treats. If you're looking for suggestions on which coffees to drink during your diet, I've compiled a few favorites here. Green beans are identified by the country of origin, followed by the region or estate where they're produced. Try to purchase from reputable roasters who've perfected light roasts. You can refer to the list of recommended beans and roasters in the Resources section for more suggestions.

MORNING

KENYAN KAROGOTO

KENYAN ICHAMAMA
ETHIOPIAN HAMBELA
ETHIOPIAN SIDAMO

These are light, East African coffees with the highest amounts of polyphenols. They will help wake you up and deliver health benefits that will improve your mood and your vascular health. Kenyan coffees are great, full-bodied waker-uppers, so they feel almost like meals. Ethiopian coffees have a zesty effervescence that offers a great midmorning punch.

AFTERNOON
ETHIOPIAN SIDAMO DECAF
MEXICAN ESMERALDA DECAF

I drink these coffees every afternoon. They're very high in CGAs, which gives me unlimited energy for my evening workouts. While most decafs have a deservedly awful reputation for taste, these are fantastic!

EVENING
COLOMBIAN HUILA EXCELSO
BRAZILIAN SITIO REZENDE

If you're one of the few who can drink a caffeinated coffee in the evening, then this is the time to enjoy slightly darker roasts. These two beans do beautifully in medium roasts. Drinking a medium-roast, high-phenol coffee after a meal will help with digestion, since it will contain the helpful melanoidins we've discussed. Latin American coffees lend themselves well to darker roasts. If you really enjoy the taste of darker roasts, then look for "lighter" dark roasts, with finish temperatures around 425 degrees, as opposed to 470 degrees, which is considered burnt by most serious roasters. Try the coffees above black, or enjoy a frothy cappuccino in place of a high-calorie dessert.

SUCCESS!

A life coach, wife, and mother of two boys from New Jersey, Marney Rohda knows how to diet. She's smart and self-aware, and incredibly disciplined, but a lack of energy while dieting made her past efforts at losing weight especially challenging. "This time, I feel really good," Marney says of the Coffee Lover's Diet. "I'm able to do all the things I'm supposed to do: take care of my kids, take care of my husband, work. I didn't have to pause my life to do the diet. The coffee made me be able to keep going."

In the past, Marney says, she'd stop working out while she was dieting, because she didn't have the energy. Then she'd try to catch up with exercise once she'd lost weight. On the Coffee Lover's Diet, she's up and at a barre class at five fifteen in the morning, several times a week. "I haven't stopped this time," she says.

Three weeks in, Marney had lost almost thirteen pounds. In addition to an energy boost, she found the coffee to be a comforting reward. The weather was beginning to get cold when she started the program. When you're only drinking smoothies, Marney says, "Coffee is warm and satisfying. It helps. Not only are you allowed to drink coffee, you're *supposed* to drink coffee. That's your medicine." The physical part, Marney says, is easy: "When you make a smoothie in the morning, and you put blueberries and kale and chia in it, you're going to feel good. It happens every time. Once you beat the mental game, the physical game is no big deal. You don't feel cranky, or low-energy, or hungry."

Well on her way to losing her goal of twenty to twenty-five pounds, feeling energized and happy, Marney found another good thing happening. She has Lyme disease, which has caused chronic eczema that leaves her skin raw and bleeding, despite the use of prescription steroid creams. Just a few weeks into her new regimen of anti-inflammatory foods and coffees, she went a week without applying any medicated cream. "My skin was a little aggravated, but it feels like no big deal. Right now I don't have a single open sore on my body," she says.

Marney's friend, Gloria Culmone, who embarked on the Coffee Lover's Diet with her, found that the coffee helped her curb her snacking habit. Hunger, thankfully, wasn't a problem for the part-time kindergarten teacher in her midforties. "I've really got to say, between chia and coffee, I'm not hungry," Gloria reports. "It was my habit to come home from work and eat junk. Mentally, I wanted to get the food. Now I go to the coffee."

As Gloria shifted from high-calorie snacks to coffee, she also made a gradual switch to drinking it black. "It took me a little bit of time. I went from cow's milk to almond milk to black," she says. Now she can enjoy three to four cups a day without any added fat or sugar.

Drinking smoothies and walking three to five miles several times a week, Gloria lost 14.5 pounds in three weeks, and aims to lose 30 more. She lists a string of improvements that makes my heart sing: "I don't get tired at work anymore. I feel energized. I physically feel like I can move differently. I feel more clear-minded. I feel healthier. Even my skin, my hair, and my nails are better, more radiant." Hooray, Gloria!

PHASE II. ACCELERATION

Because the Coffee Lover's Diet is so flexible and easy to tailor to individual needs and lifestyles, we don't prescribe a time frame for each phase. You'll know when it's time to move on. Some people strive to reach a weight goal before moving on, while others begin to feel so much better that they want to exercise more, and thus need a bit more fuel. For some, the urge to chew solid food or share meals with others initiates the transition. Depending on how much weight you want to lose and your lifestyle, an appropriate time on Phase I may be three days, or three weeks. By adding a solid meal in Phase II, you'll rev your metabolism with a careful increase of calories, added protein, hearty grains, and lots of veggies. This is the plan:

■ **TWO CHIA SMOOTHIES: ONE FOR BREAKFAST, ONE FOR LUNCH OR DINNER**

Choose any of the smoothie recipes in chapter 6, and make two servings in the morning (or at night for the following day).

■ **ONE SOLID MEAL FOR LUNCH OR DINNER**

In chapter 6 you'll find fourteen recipes for mouthwatering meals that you can make for lunch or dinner. These easy-to-follow recipes have been carefully calibrated by a nutritionist to have just the right levels of calories, fat, and protein to energize and satisfy you, while keeping your weight loss on track. Choose one meal to make for lunch or dinner.

- **COFFEES: HIGH-PHENOL COFFEES, IDEALLY BLACK, THROUGHOUT THE DAY**

    (If you're starting your diet with Phase II, see the coffee tips in Phase I.)

- **SNACKS**

    Choose a snack from our recipes, once or twice per day.

- **EXERCISE**

    Adding a solid meal may allow you to step up your exercise a bit. Add to the frequency, time, or distance of your workouts as you feel up to it.

"Every time we do this, we feel renewed, recalibrated, refreshed, and energized (not to mention pounds lighter). We've gotten so hooked that we now do Phase II at the beginning of each season to recharge ourselves. We often do a couple days at the beginning of each month, or a week if we've been feeling blah." –Chefs Mary Barber and Sara Whiteford

SUCCESS!

For those of you who know how hard it is to keep weight off when you sit at a desk for much of the day, Patrick Feeney's story is an inspiration. An American importer-exporter, Patrick spent fifteen years on the move, traveling frequently while working for a European company. The fifty-four-year-old now works in China and the Philippines, and, while he enjoys his work, he says he's spent the last three years sitting at a desk. "From a health standpoint, it's killing me," he says. "This is my fight back."

After three weeks of trying a simple, restricted-calorie diet, Patrick began the Coffee Lover's Diet. For three more weeks, he drank three chia smoothies a day, enjoyed high-phenol coffees throughout the morning, and committed to walking five miles a day. Then he shifted to Phase II. At six foot one, Patrick weighed 270 pounds when he began. After seven weeks, he had lost fifty pounds, about a pound a day. "I feel so, so much better. I feel utterly fantastic," he says. "I've lost half my girlfriend's body weight!" A trip home to the States challenged Patrick to balance family meals and celebrations with his plan, but the progress he'd made kept him on the right track. "I'm struggling with that, but I'll adapt," he reports. "Losing about a pound a day— that was so encouraging."

Another drastic improvement resulted from Patrick's efforts: a remarkable drop in his blood pressure. Before starting the diet, he went to get a new prescription for his contacts, and the technician took his blood pressure. He knew he had a family history of hypertension, but, he says, "the reading was 911." Patrick's systolic pressure, which is the top number that measures pressure in the arteries when the heart contracts, was 225. In the seven weeks that he lost fifty pounds, that number fell to 122. "Getting my blood pressure to almost a high normal without medication is a godsend," he says.

Patrick feels that there's a happy medium somewhere between Western attitudes toward health care, which he calls the take-this-pill approach, and the Eastern philosophy he's encountered that relies heavily on Chinese herbs. Losing fifty pounds and dramatically improving his blood pressure using regular exercise and superfoods like coffee and chia felt to him like "the perfect halfway spot." Having reached his initial goal of 220 pounds, he's now aiming for 200.

PHASE III. REVIVAL

Phase III is a true joy for absolutely anyone. If you're a serious dieter who's worked hard to shed weight, you'll be rewarded with a wide variety of amazingly flavorful meals, snacks, and smoothies that will not stall your progress. If you're at a healthy weight, but occasionally need to realign your eating and drinking habits, Phase III is guaranteed to revive and recharge you. Wherever you are on your journey, all the work has been done for you here; there is no guesswork regarding what to eat or how much of it. The nutrition has been vetted, recipes tested, calories counted, and there's something to fulfill any craving: savory, sweet, warm, cold, crunchy, or smooth. All you need to do is decide what you're in the mood to eat!

Because the recipes are so spectacular, we've designed Phase III to work either as a weight-loss program or a maintenance plan that you can stick with indefinitely. As you've read, choosing a smoothie, two meals, and snacks from the recipes in the following chapter will give you approximately 1,500 calories per day, which is a general guideline for weight loss. Men losing weight may need to double their snack portions to bring their intakes closer to 1,800 calories per day. I encourage you to consult your doctor and individualize your plan as needed.

If you love the recipes and the regimen, but you're ready to maintain your weight, simply add a half portion to the recipes, which will build toward a 2,000 to 2,200-calorie-per-day maintenance plan. The Mayo Clinic has an excellent online calculator that uses your weight, height, sex, and activity level to determine your calorie needs more precisely (http://www.mayoclinic.org/healthy-lifestyle/nutrition-and-healthy-eating/in-depth/calorie-calculator/itt-20084939). Be sure

BOB ARNOT, M.D.

to make this shift gradually, because suddenly adding five or six hundred extra calories per day will likely cause you to regain weight. You might begin by adding an extra snack each day for a week; add a second snack the following week; then begin to add an extra half portion of one of the meals for a few days the following week. In this way, slowly build up to your maintenance level.

- **ONE CHIA SMOOTHIE FOR BREAKFAST**

    Choose one of the smoothie recipes in chapter 6, and make one serving for breakfast.

- **TWO SOLID MEALS**

    Choose two meals from our bank of recipes to make for lunch and dinner.

- **COFFEES: HIGH-PHENOL COFFEES, IDEALLY BLACK, THROUGHOUT THE DAY**

    (See the coffee tips in Phase I.)

- **SNACKS**

    Choose a snack from our recipes, once or twice per day.

- **EXERCISE**

    Even at the weight-loss level, Phase III should give you plenty of fuel to exercise moderately. Do as much as you feel able, since exercise helps people better manage stress and avoid obsessing over food. Once you reach the maintenance plan, it's full steam ahead!

A SAMPLE DAY

7:30 A.M.	First cup of coffee: Kenyan Nyeri
8:30 A.M.	Dr. Bob's Super Smoothie, to be sipped throughout the morning
9:30 A.M.	Second coffee: Ethiopian Hambela
10:30 A.M.	Snack: a slice of whole grain bread with almond butter and jam
12:00 P.M.	Lunch: Indian lentil soup with fire-roasted tomatoes and spinach
1:30 P.M.	Third coffee: Sidamo Decaf
3:00 P.M.	Snack: plain Greek yogurt with fresh strawberries, honey, and cacao nibs
4:30 P.M.	Fourth coffee: Sidamo Decaf
5:30–7:00 P.M.	Work out
7:00 P.M.	Chipotle turkey burger with pineapple-sugar snap pea salsa

SUCCESS!

Just a few weeks into the Coffee Lover's Diet, Elaine and Roberto Torres were happy to be losing significant weight, but the husband and wife from Orlando, Florida, also experienced unanticipated results that amazed them.

Elaine's weight had fluctuated over the years and was hovering stubbornly around 200 pounds when she started the diet. Within eighteen days, she was down to 186 pounds, then quickly dropped another 3—and felt her energy level soar. "It's been life changing, getting back the energy I used to have," she says. Other times Elaine had dieted, she felt she couldn't think straight. She'd go to her desk to work and want only to take a nap. "Now I want to burn energy," she says, talking rapidly. "I want to walk the dog. I'm not getting cravings. I never feel lethargic; I feel phenomenal!"

Weeks used to pass without Elaine's venturing to the second level of their home, where the Torreses keep a treadmill and stationary bike. Now, Elaine says, she's not only willing to tackle the stairs, she walks on the treadmill for forty to forty-five minutes most days, and has begun to run for short intervals. "I'm actually running, which I've never done in my life," Elaine says. "I can actually run without feeling like I'm going to have a heart attack!"

Her husband, Roberto, dropped twenty-three pounds and, like Elaine, was determined to lose still more. Diagnosed with type 2 diabetes in 1998, Roberto has taken medication for it ever since. Enjoying his coffee, drinking chia smoothies, and eating one meal per day, Roberto also increased his exercise, walking about forty-five minutes a day on the treadmill. As the numbers on the scale fell, so did those of his fasting blood sugar. Soon he found that he no longer needed his medication. Roberto's blood sugar fell from a range of 110 to 150 with medication to a range of 95 to 102 without it. He'd never dropped below 100 with medication.

"Diabetes took my parents from me way too soon," Roberto says. "Seeing myself following in their footsteps, I decided to do something about it. It's a lifestyle choice, a decision you make and have to commit to it. I had been using diabetes medication since the age of twenty-seven, and I can tell you that not depending on my medication has been one of the most liberating experiences I have lived thus far."

Elaine says happily of her husband, "He's living proof that with diet and exercise, you can control your diabetes."

POINTERS FOR SUCCESS

As you've seen, the Coffee Lover's Diet is all about you. It's no piece of cake; it requires discipline and a huge commitment to yourself, but we promote flexibility and urge you to do what works for you. If one phase seems overwhelming, try the next one, or incorporate some of our snacks into your day, or even tackle just one or two days at a time. The idea is to come up with a plan that works for you, using our general guidelines. Return to any phase after the holidays, before bathing suit weather, or after a vacation splurge. Whenever the mood strikes, focus on yourself and reorient your diet for healthier living and a higher consciousness. You deserve it! Here are some tips to help you succeed:

- Encourage your partner, roommate, or friend to do this with you. In addition to the camaraderie, you can share the cost of the ingredients.
- Schedule this program when you have a little downtime. Too many dinner or lunch commitments can get you off track.
- Spend time in advance purchasing all the ingredients. They can be found at Whole Foods, Hannaford, Wegmans, Shaw's, Publix, and other high-end grocers, but if you don't have access to one, visit your local health food store or buy ingredients online.
- Eat organic and locally grown fruits and vegetables whenever possible, grass-fed meats, and wild fish (not farm-raised).
- Don't eat past seven thirty P.M. if possible. It's best to consume your calories earlier in the day.
- Limit alcohol consumption because it slows your metabolism and lowers inhibitions, making you more likely to overeat.

- Encourage your kids to eat what you are eating, but don't limit their intake of calories.
- Prepare items like quinoa and trail mix at the beginning of the week for easy access throughout the week.
- Make this diet work for you. All of the snacks are about 150 calories with five to ten grams of fat, so mix and match as you see fit. If you are a working parent and this seems overwhelming, eat the same snack twice a day and make your smoothies the night before. Men, double down on the snacks if you need to net closer to 1,800 calories per day.
- If you're vegetarian, substitute tofu, tempeh, seitan, or beans for meat protein.
- If you fall off the program, put it behind you pronto, and get back on board. Remember, you're human.
- Listen to your body and its needs. If you are feeling overly hungry or deprived, have a coffee or an extra snack. On the other hand, if you are starting to feel full, stop eating even if you haven't finished. Eat again when you are hungry. There is an ebb and flow that accompanies this program, and highs and lows are normal. Hang in there, as the end result will be REVIVAL!

FOR ATHLETES

Nothing aids an athlete like coffee. For me, the ability to improve my athletic performance is coffee's biggest attraction. Likewise, the most enthusiastic fans of our test brand coffees are athletes who've seen immediate improvement in their performances after drinking them. This prompted me to want to share some fueling tips from the pros for using coffee in training and in competition. First, a quick review of how coffee enhances performance:

1. Caffeine helps to liberate fatty acids for use as fuel during exercise, so that you preserve your precious muscle sugar (glycogen) stores. While burning fat is paramount to dieters, simultaneously preserving muscle sugar stores helps endurance athletes go the extra miles. In long-distance training, sugar is speed, says my coach, Hunter Allen. The higher your sugar stores, the faster you will go.

2. Caffeine and phenols are proven to increase speed and power during exercise. As icing on the cake, our own clinical trial at NCRC demonstrated that athletes who drank high-phenol caffeinated coffees experienced significant reductions in perceived exertion just a half hour into exercise. Drink coffee an hour before working out to maximize this benefit. A good guideline for dosing is 3 to 6 milligrams of caffeine per kilogram of body weight

(or 1.35 milligrams to 2.78 milligrams per pound). For instance, a 200-pound man would drink 272 to 545 milligrams of caffeine, whereas a 120-pound woman would drink 163 to 327 milligrams of caffeine. As always, be mindful of your individual tolerance (as 545 milligrams is well over the FDA recommended limit of 400 milligrams).

3. Coffee polyphenols load the blood with anti-inflammatory, antioxidant compounds, combating the oxidation of free radicals created during exercise. Soaking up those oxidants makes workouts easier and recovery faster.

FAT-BURNING MORNING TRAINING

For the last few years I've been working with world-famous cycling coach Hunter Allen, a former professional cyclist now based in Virginia. Hunter coaches me for stand-up paddling and cycling, and taught me this fat-burning technique he uses with his clients—some of the top athletes on the planet, pro cyclists and the like. The goal is to get off of sugar as a fuel, and onto fat. He does this by having them train two mornings a week after drinking coffee and skipping breakfast. "Get out there on your workout and exercise for at least two hours at a relatively low intensity, which might be considered as endurance or tempo pace," Hunter says. "At the end of two hours, make sure you eat some good complex carbs and protein to fuel you for your more intense part of the workout, coming in hour three. Get that body burning fat right from the start, and you'll be able to turn it into a fat-burning machine." Try the technique if you work out in the morning. Drink your coffee, skip breakfast, and get going. The coffee improves fat utilization right away. You'll love how lean you get, and how much better your body feels switching fuels from sugar to fat.

FUELING FOR COMPETITION

When competing, especially in endurance sports, you'll need some breakfast fuel to propel you farther and faster. Dr. Nieman helped me develop a fueling regime for my long-distance competitions in stand-up paddling, but it may also be used for other endurance sports, such as cycling, kayaking, canoeing, and hiking. (When you're testing a new fueling regime, I recommend trying it in practice, before you compete!)

- Three hours before race: high-phenol coffee
- Two hours before: light breakfast of Cream of Wheat
- One hour before: high-phenol coffee
- Ten minutes before: one large Gatorade. (Skratch and other companies also make good blends of electrolytes, glucose, and fructose. The key is to load up both the glucose and fructose transporter systems. Extensive scientific research has shown Gatorade to be very effective.)

- Forty-five minutes after start: one small Gatorade
- Every thirty minutes afterward: one small Gatorade.

In a grueling, twenty-mile open-ocean race last summer, called the Blackburn Challenge, I beat competition less than a third my age, in part by outfueling them. The body can use up to ninety grams of sugar per hour during prolonged endurance contests, while most athletes are lucky to take in fifteen grams per hour. I use this same regime for the uber-challenging thirty-two-mile world championship stand-up paddling race from Molokai to Oahu.

Remember, the Coffee Lover's Diet is engineered so that you can make it your own. Whether you're a black-coffee athlete or you're hooked on oversize, decadent coffee concoctions, whether you need to lose five pounds, fifteen, or fifty, there is a plan here for you. First, change your coffee to high-phenol beans with lighter roasts, and skip the cream and sugar. When you want a treat, try the delicious, nutritious coffee drinks found in the next chapter. Embrace the chia smoothie no matter who you are, as it's not just about staying power, but also fulfilling micronutrient hunger and calming inflammation. Then, elevate your solid meals with our flavorful, diverse recipes. Trust me, they make the best-tasting "diet" food you've ever put in your mouth. Finally, exercise! Whether you bike twenty miles or walk two, it is absolutely essential to get out there and get moving.

BOB ARNOT, M.D.

THE RECAP

1. Coffee spurs weight loss by boosting your metabolism, increasing your exercise pace, helping you burn fat, produce less fat, absorb less fat . . . you get the idea. As if that weren't enough, coffee gives you extra energy and improves your mood!

2. The chia smoothie maximizes your intake of important nutrients, giving you more of them than most Americans consume in a month. It will reduce inflammation and keep you feeling full, helping you feel better than you ever have while dieting.

3. Phase I. Initiation: Drink chia smoothies for breakfast, lunch, and dinner.

4. Phase II. Acceleration: Drink two chia smoothies and eat one solid meal, for lunch or dinner, made from our recipes in chapter 6.

5. Phase III. Revival: Drink one chia smoothie and eat two solid meals, made from our recipes in chapter 6.

6. In all phases, eat one or two snacks, but only if you're hungry. Drink high-phenol coffees black, throughout the day, choosing decaf according to your needs.

7. Exercise as you're able.

8. To maximize your exercise, drink high-phenol coffee (caffeinated if possible) an hour before you work out.

Q AND A

Q. I LOVE CREAM AND SUGAR IN MY COFFEE. HOW CAN I STOP USING THEM?

A. First, choose a lighter roast of really great beans. Good coffees have a great deal of natural sweetness, and more flavor compounds than red wines. Once you can taste those flavors, I think you'll learn to love black coffees. Second, select coffees that naturally complement healthier foods, so that you can create a magnified taste treat with good pairings. By substituting an Ethiopian Hambela and blueberries for a dark roast and cream, you'll make a doubly healthy choice. Finally, notice how much better you feel when you drink coffee this way!

Q. HOW SOON WILL I FEEL THE EFFECT OF COFFEE?

A. Caffeine takes effect within minutes and peaks in about one hour. The phenols need several hours to take effect, so you should be feeling progressively better for several hours after you drink a cup of high-phenol, black coffee. There's a long-term effect as well. The quality of the bacteria in the gut is very important to human health and can affect how much sugar and fat you absorb from meals. Phenols improve gut bacteria so that they are increasingly better absorbed. Expect a two-week loading period while the gut bacteria change, then you will feel amazing. (This

is very hard to do using other dietary measures, even probiotics.)

**Q. IF I WANT TO USE COFFEE TO BOOST MY WORKOUT, WHEN
SHOULD I DRINK IT?**

A. Drink it an hour prior to get maximum effects from the caffeine. To get maximum phenol effects, drink one cup three
hours before your workout, and another one hour before.
Many of the polyphenols are processed in the colon, so the
effect is felt a few hours after consumption.

**Q. WHAT DO YOU LIKE BEST ABOUT COFFEE WHEN YOU ARE DIET-
ING?**

A. More than anything, I love the limitless supply of energy
I get from both phenols and caffeine. I jump out of bed
and head for my coffee grinder first thing in the morning,
and at one A.M. I'm still going strong. The effect of high-
phenol coffee on mood is just phenomenal, so I always feel
great. Plus, we all fidget when we diet. We're tempted to
grab a cookie, bagel, sandwich, whatever. The careful, artisanal preparation of coffee helps you avoid temptation.
The smell of the freshly ground beans, the aroma of the
freshly brewed coffee, and the out-of-this-world taste of
artisanal coffees provide a magnificent substitute for eating. I prepare a beverage about every two hours. It's a great
time-out from work!

Q. I'VE READ THAT BREAKFAST IS A DIETER'S MOST IMPORTANT MEAL. IS IT?

A. We thought that for decades, but new studies show that it makes no difference.[9] I usually have a cup of coffee at seven A.M., nine, and eleven (some of which are decaf). This keeps me full and kills my hunger so I've had no calories though midday. At eleven thirty A.M., I make my first smoothie and nurse it through late afternoon. This gives me ultimate control over my diet.

Q. IN PHASE II OF THIS DIET, DO YOU RECOMMEND LUNCH OR DINNER?

A. First of all, eating only smoothies in Phase I is hard, so don't feel bad when you need to add a meal; doing so will keep you on track and keep your metabolism from slowing. I often do a long workout in the late afternoon, so I prefer adding lunch, so I don't go in with too few calories and bonk. I also like lunches because I like to go to bed a little hungry, as I don't want a lot of food in my stomach to disturb my sleep. If dinner makes more sense for your lifestyle, however, there's great satisfaction in feeling that you're on a roll all day with your smoothies, then enjoying a light dinner.

Q. I FIND EVENINGS THE HARDEST PART OF THE DAY TO CONTROL MY EATING. WHAT DO YOU DO?

A. First, I make sure that I have enough chia in my stomach to continue to kill my appetite. I may drink smoothies later into the day, or drink a glass of water with a couple of tablespoons of chia stirred into it. Next, I choose lean proteins for dinner. Salmon, turkey, and chicken are great, filling choices. Finally, I'll have a snack if I really must eat. My choice is often a handful of cereal, such as Kashi Oat Flakes & Blueberry Clusters. The carbs can also help you fall asleep, but do this only if you can stop at a handful.

Q. WHAT IF I HAVE HEARTBURN FROM ALL THE COFFEE AND SMOOTHIES?

A. Good question. It's easier to overload your system if you have reflux disease, in which a weak lower esophagus allows food and fluid to seep back up into your esophagus. Foremost, make sure you are following the appropriate treatment. Your doctor may recommend medicines such as Zantac or Prevacid. Heartburn poses a long-term risk of esophageal cancer, so you definitely want to treat it. Next, cut your chia intake to half a tablespoon, then gradually increase the dosage. Remember that the smoothies are meant to be sipped, not gulped. Finally, you may try letting your coffee clear your system before drinking your smoothie.

Q. CAN I HAVE TEA?

A. Sure! Green tea is much lower in overall polyphenols than coffee, but it does have highly specialized ones called catechins that have unique benefits.

CHAPTER 6

RECIPES AND PAIRINGS

RECIPES AND PAIRINGS

Welcome to the chapter that we hope you'll turn to again and again, as you prepare food and beverages that will sustain and delight you and your loved ones. This chapter combines multiple weight control resources. First, our unique recipes offer easy substitutions for the coffee drinks and foods that have led you astray from the way you want to look and feel. From coffee drinks to smoothies, snacks, lunches, and dinners, the recipes found here will make weight loss easier and more enjoyable. Second, coffee pairing, one of the hottest innovations in coffee, will help you trim hundreds of calories a day, while adding healthful foods to your diet.

Coffee drinks are some of the greatest nutritional disasters in the American diet, potentially adding hundreds of extra calories a day. These sweet treats are hard to give up, especially because they are paired with the mood boost you get from coffee. In this chapter we offer you seven incredibly delicious but totally nutritious recipes for coffee drinks that you can substitute for those dessert-like beverages, while doing something good for yourself.

In addition to the coffee drinks, you'll find nine smoothie recipes and a special tonic, fourteen snacks, and fourteen meals, every one of which has been kitchen tested and analyzed by a nutritionist. While any of the meals may be made for lunch or dinner, seven of them work particularly well when prepared ahead, so they make great lunches that you can take to work.

All of our recipes were created by Mary Barber and Sara Whiteford, who work their twin magic to consistently elevate food to its most nutritious, most delicious state. Always learning about new ingredients and new techniques, they're on the cutting edge of good food, and love sharing their discoveries and creations. For this book, they've chosen the healthiest, most natural, most nutritious ingredients, and whirled them into tantalizing combinations.

Read through these delicious recipes and choose the ones you love best, then mix and match them to suit any phase of the Coffee Lover's Diet. This is not a strict, number-crunching program, but we have provided calorie counts for all of the recipes to create a modular structure. When you're dieting, choose among the recipes so that your daily calorie total reaches roughly 1,500. Adjust as necessary to meet your personal needs. To maintain weight, move gradually toward a total of approximately 2,000 to 2,200 calories per day, or whatever the Mayo Clinic's clever personalized calorie calculator determines for you (link found on page 238). With this in mind, we've included instructions for increasing portions of the meal recipes as you shift from dieting to weight maintenance.

The recipes will help you create truly outstanding meals, but to keep you on track when you're not using them, we also offer a straightforward list of dependable foods that are healthy and weight-loss friendly. As this list helps me battle endless temptations and arms me with the nutrition I need, I call it the War Chest. You can think of it as a shopping list, or even a menu for deconstructed meals.

The War Chest is followed by a special section on pairing coffees with foods. As coffee appreciation has grown to resemble that of wine, trends in pairing unique coffees with complementary foods have exploded. Pairing is fun and creative, and vastly enhances the flavors of both food and coffee, creating a better sensory experience than either offers alone. Many people already pair coffee with cream and sugar, sometimes in wildly debilitating amounts. A sixteen-ounce serving of a popular cold, blended, caramel coffee drink, for example, has 420 calories and 15 grams of fat. We'll teach you, instead, to pair excellent coffees with great-tasting but good-for-you foods.

Now it's time to dive in. Mary and Sara have introduced each recipe for you. I hope you'll enjoy them as much as I do!

RECIPES

COFFEE DRINKS

COLD BREW CONCENTRATE

Cold brew is easy to make at home in three simple steps, without any gear. It can be done in any sort of large container (we prefer glass), a French press, or even a Mason jar. Really, if it holds coffee and water, you can cold-brew in it.

STEP 1. Measure and grind the coffee. While the perfect ratio of coffee grounds to water depends on personal taste, a good place to start is 1 cup of whole beans to 4 cups of cold water, which suits the size of a 32-ounce French press. You can double or triple these quantities depending on the size of your container. Grind the beans very coarsely. We mean it. While finer grinds offer better extraction of phenols, cold brews require a coarser grind for optimal taste. Fine grinds here will result in cloudy coffee that doesn't taste nearly as good.

STEP 2. Soak and wait (and wait, and wait . . .). Put the coffee and water in your container. The container should be deep enough to hold the coffee and water and light enough that you can pick the whole thing up to strain. Stir gently, making sure all the coffee grounds are moistened. Cover the top of your container with a lid if it has one, or cheesecloth if it doesn't. If using a French press, place the top on but don't press down on the plunger. **Let stand at room temperature for at least 12 hours and up to 18 hours.** Don't rush this. The long steep time is important for proper extraction.

STEP 3. Press/strain. If you're using a container, take the cheesecloth from the top of the container and use it to line a fine mesh sieve set over a large pitcher (or bowl or whatever else you'd like to store your cold brew in). Pour the coffee through the sieve, waiting a minute or two until the coffee has filtered through, and discard solids and cheesecloth. Add grounds to compost! For the French press, simply press down on the plunger to move grounds to the bottom. Pour into a container that can be sealed for storage.

Alternatively, you can strain your cold brew in a nut-milk bag, which is our favorite method. Simply pour steeped coffee and grounds into the open mouth of the bag and squeeze, allowing the cold brew to strain into a sealable container for storage.

Voilà. You have a cold brew. The concentrate will keep for up to two weeks covered and chilled in the fridge. It is ready to be transformed into iced coffee or any of the flavored options in this book.

HOT DRINKS

PUMPKIN GINGERBREAD LATTE

This healthy yet decadent-tasting hot toddy conjures the holiday season and makes us want to curl up beside a blazing fire. Strong brewed coffee meets pumpkin pie and gingerbread—yum! Canned pumpkin works beautifully, but if you are in the mood to bake a sugar pumpkin (not the Halloween variety), or if you have some leftover butternut squash or a sweet potato on hand, those are even better. Almond milk is wonderful, but unsweetened cashew milk works beautifully, too.

GREAT VARIATION: Try with 1 teaspoon cocoa powder. Embellish with a tablespoon of vanilla creamer for a decadent rendition, once in a while.

½ cup unsweetened vanilla almond milk

3 tablespoons pumpkin puree

1 teaspoon maple syrup

1 teaspoon pumpkin pie spice (see note)

½ teaspoon vanilla extract

2–3 drops of liquid stevia, or more to taste

1 cup strong brewed coffee (or 1–2 shots espresso)

In a saucepan, whisk together almond milk, pumpkin puree, maple syrup, pumpkin pie spice, vanilla extract, and stevia over medium heat. Alternatively, use a handheld milk frother if you have one. Add coffee and bring to a simmer. Serve. (For an extrafrothy version if you don't have a frother, blend first six ingredients in a blender until foamy just before heating.)

Makes about 1½ cups; serves 1.

CALORIES: 50

NOTE: We love the convenience of pumpkin pie spice, a warm, autumn-y blend of cinnamon, ginger, and cloves (and sometimes allspice, nutmeg, and/or mace, too) that's sold in the spice section of most supermarkets. Cloves are one of those high-phenol foods!

PEPPERMINT MOCHA LATTE

This is like a peppermint patty dipped in coffee. It is thick and frothy and voluptuous! The chocolaty flavor might feel sinful, but unsweetened cocoa powder gives you a chocolate fix without the guilt. Flavonoid-rich cocoa aids in lowering blood pressure and improving the elasticity of blood vessels. Cashew milk is widely available at grocery stores, and is a great alternative to almond and coconut milk, as it is creamy and smooth, but its flavor takes a backseat to the coffee. Along with an extra dose of phenols, the medjool dates give this drink body and sweetness that tastes truly indulgent without a speck of refined sugar. If the dates are hard, and you don't have a high-speed blender, we recommend covering them with hot water for 10–15 minutes to soften before blending.

1 cup unsweetened cashew milk
2 medjool dates, pitted
1 tablespoon cocoa powder
⅛ teaspoon peppermint extract
1 cup cold brew coffee concentrate

Combine cashew milk, dates, cocoa powder, and peppermint extract in a high-speed blender (see note). Blend until frothy and very smooth, about 1 minute. Heat coffee concentrate in small saucepan and whisk in the frothy cashew milk.

Makes about 2¼ cups; serves 2.

CALORIES: 89 PER SERVING

NOTE: Use a high-speed blender for best results for this recipe as the dates need to be fully pureed in the milk. There should not be any date flecks in the milk after it is blended.

COCONUT CREAM CAFÉ

What's not to love about a creamy coconut coffee? This is divine hot or cold. For added coconut flavor, try brewing the coffee with coconut water (see note). Don't confuse the unsweetened vanilla coconut beverage with coconut milk out of a can, which is much richer. If you aren't opposed to a little extra saturated fat with a myriad of health benefits, add 1–2 teaspoons of extra virgin coconut oil. For a supernaughty twist once in a blue moon, you can try adding a dash of coconut creamer, found in the refrigerated section of most supermarkets. Do read the labels on sweeteners and look for simple, straightforward ingredients without corn syrup.

> ¾ cup strong brewed coconut coffee (see note)
> ¾ cup unsweetened vanilla coconut milk beverage
> ¼ teaspoon coconut extract

3–5 drops vanilla stevia or 1 teaspoon maple syrup
(optional)

Combine all ingredients in a small saucepan and heat until piping hot. Dilute with water or coconut milk beverage to taste. (If you only have coconut milk out of a can on hand, use only a couple of tablespoons as it is more densely caloric.) To serve cold, simply combine all ingredients and pour over ice.

Makes about 1½ cups; serves 1.

CALORIES: 36

NOTE: Brew coffee concentrate with coconut water instead of water. It makes a wonderful nectar-like coconut coffee. Combine 1 cup coffee grounds and 2 cups coconut water in a glass jar for 8–12 hours. Strain.

COLD BLENDED DRINKS

BANANA HAZELNUT SMOOTHIE

Hazelnuts, frozen bananas, and coffee blend together to create a tantalizing trifecta. Hazelnuts, also known as filberts, are rich in dietary fiber, vitamins, and minerals, and chock-full of health-promoting phytochemicals. Throw some whole coffee beans in the mix for added texture, zing, and phenols. For extra decadence with a mocha twist, add a tablespoon of cacao powder or unsweetened cocoa powder. If your palate sways to the sweeter side, freeze ripe, freckled bananas. If you prefer less sweet, freeze the bananas when just ripe, before freckles appear.

Feel free to add to this coffee smoothie some chia or flax-seeds for added omegas and fiber, which will make it all the more satiating.

1 cup unsweetened almond milk

¾ cup cold brew coffee concentrate, room temperature or chilled

2 fresh ripe bananas, frozen and sliced

⅓ cup raw hazelnuts

6–8 ice cubes

¼ teaspoon ground cinnamon

2 tablespoons coffee beans (optional)

Combine all ingredients in blender. Blend until smooth.

Makes about 3 cups; serves 2.

CALORIES: 264 PER SERVING

POMEGRANATE RASPBERRY MOCHACCINO

Pomegranate Raspberry Mocha-licious! It's as delicious as it is healthy. Both raspberries and pomegranate juice have an array of health benefits. Both are rich sources of vitamin C and antioxidants, not to mention fiber and anti-inflammatory properties. Some studies show that eating pomegranate seeds or drinking pomegranate juice can help protect against diseases, like certain cancers and Alzheimer's. Almond butter is chock-full of healthy fats and fiber. Cashew butter works wonders, too. Cheers to healthy made delicious!

1¼ cups unsweetened almond milk

¼ cup pomegranate juice

1 cup fresh or frozen raspberries

2 tablespoons almond butter

2 tablespoons cacao powder or unsweetened cocoa powder

4 concentrated cold brew coffee ice cubes (see tip opposite)

10–15 drops stevia

Combine all ingredients in blender and blend until smooth. Start with 10 drops of stevia and add more to taste.

Makes about 2 ½ cups; serves 2.

BOB ARNOT, M.D.

CALORIES: 214 PER SERVING

TIP: Freeze concentrated cold-brewed coffee in ice cube trays for 4–8 hours. Store in a sealable bag for several weeks at a time.

BLUEBERRY POMEGRANATE FRAPPE

Blueberries, pomegranate juice, and coffee? Yep. It's delicious and the antioxidant content is off the hook. The blueberries' fiber, potassium, folate, vitamin C, vitamin B$_6$, and phytonutrients, coupled with a lack of cholesterol, all support heart health. (Wild Alaskan blueberries, in particular, are among the very highest-scoring foods for phenols.) Pair with pomegranate juice, and your heart will be so happy. For variety, try substituting unsweetened frozen açai for the blueberries. Raw cashews give body to this frappe and add a punch of vitamins, minerals, and antioxidants. The yogurt provides probiotics, which promote healthy digestion. Blueberry kefir, another probiotic-rich option, could substitute for yogurt if you have it on hand. Drink to your health!

½ cup cold brew coffee concentrate

¼ cup pomegranate juice

1 6-ounce container low-fat blueberry yogurt

2 tablespoons raw cashews

1½ cups frozen blueberries

½ teaspoon ground cinnamon

handful of ice cubes

3–5 drops stevia, or ½ teaspoon maple syrup
   (optional)

Combine coffee, pomegranate juice, yogurt, and cashews in a blender. Blend until smooth. Add blueberries, cinnamon, ice cubes, and stevia or maple syrup, if using. Blend until smooth and adjust sweetness with more stevia to taste.

Makes about 2½ cups; serves 2.

CALORIES: 202 PER SERVING

CARDAMOM CARAMEL BLENDED ICED COFFEE

This frothy, creamy date-caramel concoction has a healthy lick of salt and cardamom! It is voluptuous, sweet, and creamy, without an ounce of refined sugar or dairy. Medjool dates, known as the king of dates, bring on body, natural caramel-like sweetness, and a healthy dose of nutrition. They are full of soluble and insoluble fiber, amino acids, and an array of healthy minerals. For added sweetness, use a drop of vanilla stevia. Cardamom is divine, and if you aren't familiar with it, we urge you to give it a try. For convenience, buy it ground, instead of in whole pod form. Cinnamon or pumpkin pie spice make a fine substitute if you don't care for the cardamom.

1 cup unsweetened almond milk

4 medjool dates, pitted (scant ¼ cup)

1 cup cold brew coffee concentrate, chilled

1 teaspoon vanilla extract

⅛ teaspoon fine sea salt

⅛ teaspoon ground cardamom, plus more if desired

8–10 ice cubes

1–3 drops vanilla stevia, to taste (optional)

Combine almond milk (or coconut milk beverage if preferred) and dates in a blender. Starting on low and graduating to high speed, blend until the dates are fully incorporated and milk is completely smooth. Add coffee, vanilla extract, sea salt, cardamom, and ice cubes. Blend until frothy. Season to taste with more cardamom if desired. Add more ice to dilute sweetness, if desired. To increase sweetness, add a couple of drops of stevia to taste.

Makes about 3 cups; serves 2.

CALORIES: 56 PER SERVING

NOTE: Only Dr. Bob's Super Smoothie includes chia in the recipe, but you can add it to all the rest. Adding 2 tablespoons of chia to each recipe (and a bit more liquid) will give them about 140 additional calories. We prefer to keep our smoothies on the thinner side, and stir chia into a glass of water, or water cut with juice, or the lemon tonic recipe that follows the smoothies. It's fine to drink your chia on the side, but don't skip it; it's the key to feeling full and getting the nutrition you need.

You'll see that the smoothie recipes vary in calorie totals. Multiply these recipes as you like, and add to snacks and/or meals, to reach your targeted number of calories per day.

DR. BOB'S SUPER SMOOTHIE

1 cup water

2–4 tablespoons chia

½ cup plain, nonfat Greek yogurt (almond and coconut milk are good substitutes)

½ cup frozen blueberries

½ cup frozen cantaloupe

½ banana

3 cups chopped, stemmed, frozen kale leaves

½ cup frozen spinach

1 teaspoon wild honey, or to taste (Make it taste good, so you'll drink it!)

Combine the water, chia, yogurt, blueberries, cantaloupe, banana, kale, spinach, and honey in a blender. Blend until smooth.

NOTE: Because chia absorbs liquid to form a gel in the stomach, which helps you feel full for hours, eating too much of it too fast can make you feel bloated or give you reflux. If you're new to chia, start with a tablespoon and work your way up as your body adjusts to it.

Makes about 3 cups.

CALORIES: 393

KALE CARROT PEAR GINGER

Warning: You may fall in love with this smoothie even if you aren't a kale lover. We have served this to people who claimed they hate kale, and received rave reviews. The prominent flavors of the sweet carrot juice, tangy pear, and puckery lemon override the earthy, cruciferous kale. This smoothie is, however, great with spinach, romaine, or any premixed greens as an alternative. We have even made this smoothie with a ½ cup of quartered brussel sprouts. The almonds add some good fats that will keep you satiated throughout the day.

    1½ cups fresh pressed organic carrot juice
    ½ cup water
    1 cup firmly packed chopped kale leaves, stems
        removed
    1 small diced pear
    ¼ cup raw almonds
    1 tablespoon lemon juice
    ¼ teaspoon chopped ginger, plus more to taste

Combine the carrot juice, water, kale, pear, almonds, lemon juice, and ginger in a blender. Blend until smooth.

Makes about 3 cups.

CALORIES: 255

TOMATO MANGO CILANTRO JALAPENO

We are smitten with this Southwestern-inspired gazpacho blend, and we love it morning, noon, or night. Just because it's more savory than sweet, don't count this "souper" smoothie out for breakfast. The cilantro and jalapeno pair beautifully with the sweetness of mango, but if you aren't a cilantro lover, try basil, and cantaloupe works nicely as an alternative to the mango. This smoothie is at its best when tomatoes are at their peak. Sweet 100s are our favorite, but globe tomatoes work well.

2½ cups cherry tomatoes

1 medium carrot, peeled and roughly chopped

¾ cup roughly chopped red pepper

¾ cup roughly chopped mango

3 tablespoons chopped red onion

1 tablespoon lemon juice

2 teaspoons good extra virgin olive oil

¼ cup cilantro

1 teaspoon chopped jalapeno

½ teaspoon sea salt, plus more to taste

freshly ground pepper

Place all ingredients in a food processor fitted with a metal blade attachment. (If you don't have a food processor, a blender will work.) Season to taste with more sea salt and pepper or jalapeno.

Makes about 2½ cups.

CALORIES: 138

COCONUT MANGO BANANA SPINACH

If drinking green smoothies is beyond your comfort zone, try initiating yourself into the world of green elixirs with this one. The trio of blended coconut, mango, and banana is so captivating to the senses that the mild taste of the chlorophyll-rich spinach fades seamlessly into the background. Besides the beautiful color that the spinach imparts, it's hard to detect that an immune-boosting spinach salad has slipped into your smoothie. Add some protein-rich pumpkin seeds, as they are nutritional powerhouses with magnesium, manganese, copper, zinc, and an array of antioxidants. Use fresh or frozen fruit, depending on whether you want an icy cold or a room-temp smoothie.

1½ cups coconut water
1 cup mango, fresh or frozen
1 small banana, fresh or frozen
2 cups firmly packed spinach
3 tablespoons pumpkin seeds

Combine the coconut water, mango, banana, spinach, and pumpkin seeds in a blender. Blend until smooth.

Makes about 3 cups.

CALORIES: 232

BOB ARNOT, M.D.

GRAPEFRUIT AVOCADO CILANTRO MINT

This blend is truly one of our very faves. It may sound way out there. Grapefruit and cilantro? Trust us. This one is way, way, way delicious for those who love grapefruit, which is low in calories, full of nutrients, and an excellent source of carotenoids and vitamin C. If you aren't hip to cilantro, skip it, and if you prefer oranges to grapefruits, substitute with navel oranges when they are in season.

    1 cup fresh-pressed apple juice
    1 cup grapefruit sections (see note), and any extra
        grapefruit juice
    1 cup mint
    ½ small avocado
    ½ cup cilantro
    ½ cup water

Combine the apple juice, grapefruit (plus any extra grapefruit juice), mint, avocado, cilantro, and water in a blender. Blend until smooth.

NOTE: This smoothie is best when the grapefruit is sectioned from the white pith. If you cut it more like an apple, discarding only the "core" pith, the smoothie will be on the bitter side.

Makes about 3 cups.

CALORIES: 185

PINEAPPLE MINT SPINACH CUCUMBER

Lean, clean, and green, this combination is a refreshing and satisfying meal replacement. Sweet and delightfully tart pineapple; crisp, hydrating cucumbers; and refreshing mint play off each other so synergistically that the yum factor tops the charts. Pineapple is full of vitamins and soluble and insoluble fiber, while hemp seeds add a healthy dose of omega-3s, protein, and fiber. These mild little seeds add a decadent nuttiness to the overall good taste of the smoothie, while the antioxidant-rich spinach adds a subtle creaminess and a bright green essence.

¾ cup cucumber

1 cup fresh-pressed apple juice

1 cup chopped fresh pineapple, chilled or frozen

1 cup spinach leaves

½ cup firmly packed mint leaves

2 tablespoons hemp seeds

a few ice cubes (optional)

Combine cucumber, apple juice, pineapple, spinach, mint, hemp seeds, and ice in a blender. Blend until smooth.

Makes about 3 cups.

CALORIES: 171

AÇAI RASPBERRY BLUEBERRY BANANA

This symphony of blended berries with an accent of banana delivers outstanding health benefits. Think antioxidants, omega fats, protein, and fiber, and raise your glass to great-tasting nutrition. We recommend trying some of the different brands of açai juices on the market, as each has its own distinct berry-cocoa flavor. Bear in mind that the blueberries and bananas contain pectin, which is a natural thickener, so this smoothie will thicken significantly over time. We recommend drinking it immediately. Or pull out a spoon!

1 cup açai juice

1¼ cups blueberries, fresh or frozen

¾ cup frozen raspberries

1 fresh ripe banana

¼ cup raw cashews

Combine the açai juice, blueberries, raspberries, banana, and cashews in the blender. Blend until smooth.

Makes about 2½ cups.

CALORIES: 361

COCONUT STRAWBERRY APPLE ALMOND

This chunky, ambrosia-like smoothie is fit for the gods, it is so divine! Whether served in a bowl or a glass, a spoon is required. If you eat it for breakfast, you may never go back to dry cereal again. Coconut water is an isotonic electrolyte-rich beverage that is a wonderful complement to the phenol-packed strawberries and apple. A dollop of probiotic-rich Greek yogurt transforms this ambrosia into a creamy treat, while raw almonds add a crunchy rich texture with healthy fats, fiber, protein, magnesium, and vitamin E.

¾ cup coconut water
1 cup fresh strawberries
1 cup diced red apple, such as Fuji
½ cup plain 2 percent Greek yogurt
¼ cup raw almonds, preferably soaked and drained
3 tablespoons unsweetened coconut flakes

½ teaspoon vanilla extract

coconut extract (optional)

a few drops of stevia (optional)

Add all ingredients and pulse a few times, keeping the mixture chunky. Serve with a spoon.

Makes about 2 cups.

CALORIES: 312

CARROT BEET ARUGULA

One of our all-time favorite salad combinations is peppery arugula with beets, apples, and walnuts. Delicious! When we decided to put these complementary ingredients in the blender, a hard-to-beet salad smoothie was born. Arugula, also known as salad rocket, is a rich source of certain phytochemicals that have been shown to combat cancer-causing elements. Paired with nutritionally dense carrot juice and beets, and omega-3-filled walnuts, it will make you feel charged and alive!

1½ cups fresh pressed carrot juice

½ cup water

1 cup firmly packed arugula leaves

½ cup grated raw beets

½ red apple, core removed and roughly chopped

2 tablespoons raw walnuts

2 tablespoons lemon juice

1 teaspoon flax oil or olive oil

Combine the carrot juice, water, arugula, beets, apple, walnuts, lemon juice, and flax oil or olive oil in a blender. Blend until smooth.

Makes about 3 cups.

CALORIES: 184

LEMON REVIVAL TONIC

If hunger pangs creep up on you, try this yummy tonic, cold or hot. Satisfying and easy to make, this elixir is a lifesaver during periods of calorie restriction. It can be energizing before a workout or whenever your energy fades; it is also a warming tonic before bed and an awakening liver-cleanser first thing in the morning. We recommend 1–2 cups per day as needed. You can make a big batch ahead of time.

2 cups water

1 tablespoon maple syrup

juice of one lemon (about 1 tablespoon)

dash of cayenne

Mix all ingredients. For hot tonic, boil the water and add remaining ingredients.

Variations:

1. 1 teaspoon chopped ginger to aid digestion
2. 10 mint leaves, crushed in your hand, for fresh breath
3. ½ teaspoon vanilla extract for the vanilla lover
4. 1 teaspoon elderberry syrup brings mega polyphenols for an immunity boost (if adding, reduce maple syrup by 1 teaspoon)
5. ¼ teaspoon ground turmeric is anti-inflammatory
6. 1 tablespoon flax meal or ground chia seeds stirred into the mix right before drinking will add extra fiber and reduce appetite

GREEK YOGURT WITH STRAWBERRIES AND SPROUTED GRANOLA

With a thicker texture, fewer carbohydrates, less sugar, and more protein than regular yogurt, Greek yogurt makes a delectable breakfast. Made by separating out the whey, this creamy delight pairs beautifully with phenol-rich strawberries and low-fat, sprouted granola. (Sprouted foods aid digestion.) Your taste buds will be charmed and your belly satiated for several hours. For variety, try any type of berry as a substitute. Read the labels on granola packages, as some brands are superhigh in fat and calories. Look for a granola that has 3 grams of fat or less per serving and 5 grams or less sugar, such as KIND.

½ cup 2 percent Greek yogurt or kefir
½ cup low-fat sprouted granola
½ cup chopped strawberries
dash of cinnamon

Combine in a bowl and enjoy!

CALORIES: 291

CORN TORTILLAS WITH EGG WHITES, BLACK BEANS, AND CHERRY TOMATOES

Smoothies are great, but sometimes you'll want to live by the axiom "Eat breakfast like a king, lunch like a queen, and dinner like a pauper." There is wisdom in the saying. Not only do you get a wide variety of nutrition in this medley early in the day, but also you get nutrient-dense calories that will help prevent you from overeating at night. Cheers to a protein-enhanced version of scrambled eggs, embellished with protein and fiber-rich beans, vitamin C–rich tomatoes, and sprouted corn tortillas. Oh, did we the mention the chlorophyll-kissed basil? That's optional, but we highly recommend it!

    1 egg plus 2 egg whites
    1 tablespoon water
    fine sea salt
    freshly ground pepper
    1 teaspoon ghee (see note) or olive oil
    1 tablespoon parmesan cheese
    2 6-inch corn tortillas, preferably sprouted (see
        note)
    ¼ cup black beans
    ¼ cup cherry tomatoes, cut in half
    fresh torn basil and/or hot sauce

Whisk together eggs, water, and a pinch of fine sea salt and freshly ground pepper in small bowl with a fork. Heat ghee or olive oil in a nonstick pan over medium heat. Add egg mixture, followed by the cheese, and cook for a minute or so until desired consistency. Warm tortillas by dragging them back and forth directly (using tongs) over a gas flame, until warm and slightly charred. (Alternatively, heat in a microwave or toaster oven.) Divide scramble, black beans, and cherry tomatoes equally between the tortillas. Top with torn basil and/or hot sauce.

NOTE: Ghee, or clarified butter, is a must in our kitchen. We keep it on hand for many reasons, mainly for its rich, nutty taste and high smoke point, but also for its range of health benefits. Ghee has a unique nutrition profile as it has no lactose or casein. Those who are lactose- or casein-sensitive can use ghee, because these allergens are removed. If you've been told to stay away from dairy and butter, try experimenting with ghee made from grass-fed cows' butter.

NOTE ON SPROUTED FOODS: The process of germination changes the composition of grain and seeds in numerous ways. It not only amps the vitamin content, but it neutralizes phytic acid, a substance in grains that inhibits absorption of nutrients. Sprouting can also help with digestion, so it's a win-win. Look for sprouted foods, raw and baked. The corn tortillas are generally in the refrigerated and/or frozen sections of grocery stores.

CALORIES: 217

SNACKS

GRANOLA WITH BLUEBERRIES AND AÇAI

This is a simple and satisfying snack loaded with phenols. Açai's unique berry-cocoa flavor gives this snack an enhanced flavor twist. If you don't have açai on hand, you can fork-smash an extra ¼ cup of blueberries as a substitute. Feel free to use strawberries, raspberries, or blackberries in place of the "blues" if you want to shake things up a bit.

    ¼ cup low-fat granola
    ⅓ cup blueberries, or berries of choice
    ½ of one 3.5-ounce unsweetened frozen açai
        smoothie pack (slightly thawed)
    1–3 drops of stevia, to taste

Mix ingredients together in a bowl. Start with a little stevia and add more to taste. A little goes a long way. In case you missed the recipe for Greek yogurt with granola and strawberries, please note that there are many types of granola on the market these days that will sabotage weight loss. Look for brands, such as KIND, that have 3 grams of fat per serving or less, and 5 grams or less of sugar. If you can find sprouted granola, that is ideal.

CALORIES: 146

HUMMUS WITH CARROT STICKS

This crunchy-meets-creamy combo is an ideal snack when you are on the go and hunger pangs strike! Feel free to use broccoli, sugar snap peas, red peppers, or jicama sticks for variety. We're all about homemade, from-scratch cooking. That being said, we purchase store-bought hummus when we need a quick, on-the-fly snack. We often add a fresh squeeze of lemon juice and a dash of fresh cumin, or a little cilantro and/or fresh mint to the store-bought version if we feel inspired.

⅓ cup hummus
1 medium carrot, peeled and cut into sticks

Dip away!

CALORIES: 143

CANTALOUPE AND COTTAGE CHEESE

If you haven't discovered this brilliant combo, we urge you to try it; the pairing goes together like peanut butter and jelly. Cottage cheese also pairs beautifully with stone fruits such as nectarines and peaches. Cantaloupe scores well for potassium, as well as for a host of B vitamins (B_1, B_3, B_6, and folate), vitamin K, magnesium, and fiber. Cottage cheese will bolster your protein intake and, surprisingly, your electrolyte levels.

> 3 medium wedges cantaloupe (1 wedge = 1/8 medium melon)
> ½ cup 1 percent cottage cheese

Chop cantaloupe into bite-size pieces and put in a bowl with cottage cheese.

CALORIES: 152

HANDFUL OF RAW ALMONDS

Raw almonds are so yummy, so simple, and so satiating, they feel like the perfect snack food. We recommend raw almonds, rather than roasted, as raw are more nutrient dense. During the roasting process, heat destroys the vitamins. Think over-cooked veggies. We are fans of soaking almonds overnight, but do this only if you have the bandwidth to think ahead. The soaking process releases phytic acids in the almonds, which makes them more digestible. If you really want to amp your health game, peel those babies to make them even more di-gestible!

20 raw almonds

If you have time, soak nuts in water overnight or even for a few hours. Rinse and drain. Peel only if time permits.

CALORIES: 138

BROWN RICE CAKE WITH CASHEW BUTTER AND SMASHED BLUEBERRIES

Cashew butter and smashed blueberries on a crispy brown rice cake makes for a supersatisfying snack. Invest in a few nut butters and store them in the refrigerator at home or at work. Mix and match according to your taste preference. Cashew butter delights, as do other nut but-ters such as walnut, pecan, peanut, and almond. Seed butters, such as sunflower butter and tahini, are also nutritious and delicious. If you're not in love with blueberries, any berry will do.

    1 brown rice cake
    2 teaspoons raw cashew butter
    2 tablespoons blueberries, smashed
    2 teaspoons raw honey (see note)

NOTE: Choose raw honey because it contains all the pollen, enzymes, and other micronutrients that are filtered and destroyed when honey is heated and processed.

CALORIES: 152

WHOLE WHEAT TOAST WITH ALMOND BUTTER, HONEY, AND COCOA

We just gave the age-old PB&J a healthy makeover. Leave behind the white bread with "Jif and jam," and look instead for sprouted whole wheat bread, raw almond butter (ideally sprouted if available), and raw, unpasteurized honey. If you're a chocolate lover looking for a little variety, add a dusting of cocoa powder, or cacao nibs if you have them handy. This little bit is far from reckless; plus, chocolate is loaded with phenols. It will not only put you in a good mood, but can bolster your health as well.

1 slice sprouted whole grain bread

2 teaspoons raw almond butter

1 teaspoon raw honey

pinch of unsweetened cocoa powder or cacao nibs
(optional)

Toast 1 slice of whole wheat bread. Top with almond butter, honey, and cocoa powder or cacao nibs, if desired.

CALORIES: 151

TRAIL MIX

This trail mix has zing! We dare you to add whole high-phenol coffee beans and cacao nibs, too. The double-down crunch not only delights the palate and promotes a healthy immune system, but you may feel compelled to run stairs after downing this mix. Containing health-promoting raisins, sunflower seeds, walnuts, and pumpkin seeds, this snack is ultradelicious, ultrasatisfying, and ultrahealthy! Trust us, you'll be challenged to eat no more than ¼ cup.

1 cup golden raisins

¼ cup sunflower seeds

¼ cup raw walnuts

¼ cup pumpkin seeds

⅛ cup cacao nibs

⅛ cup coffee beans

Mix all ingredients in a small bowl. Store in an airtight container.

Serving size: ¼ cup

CALORIES: 137

STRAWBERRIES WITH YOGURT, HONEY, AND CACAO NIBS

The combination of fresh strawberries and yogurt with a drizzle of honey and an unexpected sprinkle of crunchy cacao nibs will so dazzle your taste buds, you may not notice the boost it will give your immune system. We all know that strawberries pack a wallop of vitamin C, but it's the free radical–fighting compounds, called anthocyanins, that are the true rock-star health components of strawberries. Anthocyanins are anticarcinogenic; the yogurt provides a hit of probiotics, essential for gut health; and chocolate lovers, rejoice, because cacao nibs are chock-full of immune-boosting goodness.

½ cup whole strawberries

½ cup 2 percent Greek yogurt

1 teaspoon raw honey

1 teaspoon cacao nibs

Place the strawberries, yogurt, a drizzle of honey, and cacao nibs in a bowl. Voilà!

CALORIES: 162

CURRIED EGG SALAD

This is a tasty and satisfying, protein-rich snack that can hang in the fridge for up to three days, so make a double or triple batch on a Sunday afternoon when you have a few minutes, and you'll be set for snacks throughout the week. Add a dash of hot sauce if you like. A slice of tomato is delicious on top. If you want to swap out the rice cake, whole wheat toast or half of a pita makes a delicious alternative.

1 hard-boiled egg, plus one egg white, mashed

3 tablespoons 1 percent cottage cheese

1 teaspoon Dijon mustard

a dash of curry powder

sea salt

ground pepper

1 brown rice cake

Combine ingredients in a bowl and spread atop rice cake.

CALORIES: 155

TURKEY AVOCADO ROLL

Think turkey club without the bread and the bacon! You really aren't missing a thing. Roll some thin turkey slices with a couple of skinny slices of avocado, some cherry tomato halves, and basil leaves, and you are rockin' and rollin'. Hold the yellow mustard, and go with any whole grain or Dijon mustard. Take it with you as an easy, on-the-go snack anytime. We like to keep a package of turkey on hand at work, as well as avocados and tomatoes. Basil is a delicious accoutrement, but don't worry if you don't have it available. A handful of any greens works perfectly. If you get in a pinch for lunch, eat three of these.

2 ounces sliced turkey (2 slices)

1 teaspoon whole grain mustard

¼ avocado

2 tablespoons chopped cherry tomatoes

whole basil leaves for garnish

Lay the 2 turkey slices side by side. Season with salt and pepper. Spread each turkey slice with ½ teaspoon mustard. Cut the avocado quarter into thin slices. Place avocado slices on the turkey. Divide the tomatoes between the two portions of turkey. Garnish with basil leaves and roll.

CALORIES: 139

SALMON SALAD TACO WITH ARUGULA AND DILL

If you fancy tuna salad, we bet you'll love this light and flavorful salmon wrap, punctuated with a zing of lemon pepper, fresh dill, and spicy arugula. This version is lower in saturated fat and less caloric than traditional, made-with-mayo tuna salad because we slipped in a touch of Greek yogurt in its place. You can thank yourself for the added boost of anti-inflammatory omega-3s in the salmon.

3 ounces prepackaged salmon

2 tablespoons 2 percent plain Greek yogurt

1 tablespoon red onion, finely chopped

½ teaspoon fresh chopped dill or ⅛ teaspoon dried
   dill

¼ teaspoon lemon pepper

1 6-inch corn tortilla, preferably sprouted

⅓ cup arugula

thin slice of tomato (optional)

Fork-smash the salmon in a small bowl. Add yogurt, red onion, dill, and lemon pepper, and stir to combine. Season with salt and more lemon pepper to taste, if desired.

Warm tortilla over a gas flame for about 30 seconds, flipping with tongs frequently until warm and slightly brown on the edges, but malleable. Alternatively, warm in the microwave. Place warm tortilla on a flat surface. Top with arugula and tomato, if using. Place salmon salad in the center of the tortilla. Fold up taco-style and eat immediately. Note: The salad can be made ahead of time. Assemble taco just before serving.

CALORIES: 140

AVOCADO WITH LIME AND SALT

We think of the avocado as a perfect food. It is high in fiber, has a healthy dose of potassium, is loaded with good fat (the monounsaturated kind)—and this is just the short list. Above all else, it's yummy and simple to prepare, and it can be spruced up in all sorts of ways. We suggest lime juice in this throw-together snack. Think guacamole without all the chopping. Feel free to add a little cumin or coriander, some cilantro leaves, or whatever suits your fancy. White balsamic is a great alternative to the lime, as is seasoned rice vinegar.

½ small avocado, pit removed

squeeze of fresh lime juice

pinch of fine sea salt

pinch of freshly ground pepper

Score the flesh of the avocado with a small knife. Be careful to avoid cutting through the skin. Squeeze lime over the avocado and season with salt and pepper. Eat out of the avocado with a spoon. No dish required!

CALORIES: 163

BANANA WITH SUNFLOWER SEED BUTTER

We've always loved bananas with some sort of nut or seed butter, so it's nice knowing that nearly all types of nuts and seeds provide healthy sources of essential fatty acids. This combo is a great choice when you're flying out the door, late to work or the gym. Although we like sunflower butter for the sake of variety, any type will do; we keep several nut butters in the fridge to slather over bananas or apples or celery. Cashew, walnut, and almond butters are good for starters, then branch out from there. They all have slightly different nutritional profiles, so shaking up your routine means shaking up your vitamin intake.

½ banana, peeled
1 tablespoon seed or nut butter

Cut a banana in half, slice it lengthwise, and spread with seed or nut butter. Reassemble if you like, or eat each slice separately. Or simply place a little portion of the nut butter on each bite, peeling the banana as you go.

CALORIES: 151

SOUTHWEST TORTILLA ROLL WITH CHICKEN AND BLACK BEANS

A tasty wrap can be assembled in minutes for a quick snack on the go. We often use chicken as a lean protein source, but if we have some smoked tofu on hand, it makes a great vegan substitute. Think of this roll as a starting point and feel free to embellish. If you have fresh herbs, cilantro or basil complement well. Red or green onions add great punch, too. This roll can be preassembled several hours in advance for a mid-morning or afternoon snack.

1 6-inch corn tortilla, preferably sprouted

¼ cup black beans, smashed

1 tablespoon salsa

1 ounce sliced chicken, or 1 slice baked tofu cut thinly

1 tablespoon fresh cilantro

dash ground cumin

dash hot sauce (optional)

Warm tortilla over a gas flame for about 30 seconds, flipping with tongs frequently until warm and slightly brown on the edges, but malleable. Alternatively, warm in the microwave. Place on flat surface. Spread mashed black beans over the warm tortilla and add salsa, followed by chicken, cilantro, cumin, and hot sauce, if desired. Roll up the tortilla and enjoy.

CALORIES: 140

LUNCHES

NOTE: For all meals, when following a weight maintenance plan, cut the recipe in half, and add that amount to the measurements that follow.

CURRIED CHICKEN SALAD WITH WHOLE WHEAT PITA

Curried chicken salad is one of those universally adored dishes that is not always friendly to the waistline. We lightened it up with some 2 percent Greek yogurt and chopped broccoli. With a little mango chutney, some fresh cilantro, and a little twang from the combo of fresh lemon juice and raisins, this dish will leave you utterly satisfied. We bet you won't even miss the extra mayo.

5 ounces boneless, skinless chicken breast, from
    roasted chicken, chopped

3 tablespoons raisins

½ cup chopped broccoli florets

3 tablespoons chopped green onion, white part only

1 tablespoon mayonnaise

3 tablespoons 2 percent plain Greek yogurt

1 tablespoon mango chutney

1 tablespoon fresh lemon juice

1 tablespoon chopped fresh cilantro (optional)

½ teaspoon curry powder

¼ teaspoon sea salt

pinch of black pepper

2 whole wheat pita rounds, top few inches of the crust
    removed to create an opening

Preheat oven to 350 degrees. Cut chicken breast into ½-inch cubes and place in a medium bowl. Add raisins, broccoli florets, green onion, mayonnaise, yogurt, chutney, lemon juice, cilantro, curry powder, salt, and pepper. Mix until combined. Heat pita in oven. Season chicken salad to taste with more salt, pepper, and lemon juice. Add ¾ cup chicken salad to each pita pocket and serve.

Serves 2 (¾ cup per serving).

CALORIES: 515 PER SERVING

VEGGIE CHILI

This quickie chili is great weeknight fare, and perfect for a take-to-work lunch, as it's best made several hours in advance and tastes even better the next day. Make it on a Sunday night for easy meals throughout the week. If you are new to veggie chili, and not used to the idea of the vegetarian "crumbles," we encourage you to give them a try! We serve this dish to our families as chili (not veggie chili) and they have never once questioned the meat source. They have no idea they are eating a 100 percent plant-protein dinner! If you still aren't persuaded, substitute about 6 ounces cooked lean ground turkey or a cup of drained beans in lieu of the veggie crumbles.

1½ cups uncooked long-grain brown rice

1 tablespoon olive oil

1 cup onion, chopped

1 cup celery, chopped (about 1 stalk)

1 cup red bell pepper, chopped

1 tablespoon minced garlic

½ cup water, divided

1 teaspoon dried oregano

1 teaspoon ground cumin

½ teaspoon fine salt

1 15-ounce can crushed fire-roasted tomatoes

1 15-ounce can black beans, liquid included

1 cup (6 ounces) vegetarian crumbles (suggested
    brand: Beyond Beef)

1 tablespoon chili powder

2 teaspoons maple syrup

1 teaspoon smoked paprika

Optional: Garnish each serving with a little chopped
    cilantro (2 teaspoons per serving), hot sauce,
    and/or 1 tablespoon 2 percent Greek yogurt (adds
    17 calories).

Prepare rice according to package directions. (You may have a little more rice than you will need as each serving is ¾ cup cooked rice, and 1½ cups uncooked rice may yield more).

Heat the olive oil in a medium pot over medium heat. Stir in the onion, celery, red pepper, garlic, ¼ cup water, oregano, cumin, and salt. Cook over medium heat, stirring frequently, until vegetables are tender, 10–15 minutes. Add the fire-roasted tomatoes, black beans (with liquid), vegetarian crumbles, chili powder, maple syrup, smoked paprika, and remaining ¼ cup water. Add more salt to taste. Reduce heat to low, cover pot, leaving a small crack, and simmer 15–20 minutes. Adjust seasonings again with more salt and chili powder or smoked paprika to taste. Serve over rice with optional garnish.

Serves 4 (1 cup chili per serving with ¾ cup cooked rice).

CALORIES: 500 PER SERVING

TUNA SALAD WITH GREEN APPLE AND DILL ON SANDWICH THINS

Green apple, dried cranberries, and fresh dill add an unexpected twist to traditional tuna salad. This version has little mayo and no relish, and we promise you won't miss them at all. Canned tuna truly comes to life in a whole new way with all the crunch coming from the apple, the celery, and the red onion, and the fresh dill is punctuated by the tartness of the lemon and the cranberries. Superb!

FOR THE SALAD:

2 tablespoons dried cranberries

1 5-ounce can tuna in water, drained thoroughly

⅓ cup celery, finely chopped

⅓ cup green apple, finely chopped

2 tablespoons chopped red onion

1½ tablespoons chopped dill

2 tablespoons 2 percent Greek yogurt

1½ tablespoons mayonnaise

1 tablespoon fresh lemon juice

1 teaspoon Dijon mustard

⅛ teaspoon fine sea salt

pinch freshly ground pepper

FOR ASSEMBLY:

2 whole wheat sandwich thins, toasted

1 small avocado, cut in half, pit removed

Soak cranberries in hot water and set aside to soften. Add drained tuna, celery, apple, red onion, dill, yogurt, mayonnaise, lemon juice, mustard, salt, and pepper in a bowl. Stir until ingredients are combined. Drain cranberries and add to the tuna mixture. Stir until combined. Season to taste with salt, pepper, and lemon juice. Toast 2 sandwich thins.

Fork-smash ½ of the avocado on the bottom of each thin, and divide tuna salad on top. Enjoy!

Serves 2 (¾ cup per serving).

CALORIES: 493 PER SERVING

GREEK SALAD WITH GRILLED CHICKEN

Greek salad is naturally suited for the health-conscious eater, as it is predominantly crunchy veggies with a light red wine vinaigrette, embellished with feta and black olives. We seek the oil-cured ones in the olive bars, but Kalamata olives work great as well. Use what you like (if green olives are your thing, they'll do fine as well). We recommend making the vinaigrette and even chopping the veggies a day in advance for quick and easy weeknight assembly.

FOR THE VINAIGRETTE:

¼ cup good red wine vinegar

1 teaspoon minced garlic (1 clove)

½ teaspoon dried oregano

½ teaspoon Dijon mustard

¼ teaspoon kosher salt

⅛ teaspoon freshly ground black pepper

¼ cup good olive oil

FOR THE SALAD:

1 cup hothouse cucumber, unpeeled, seeded, and
   sliced ¼-inch thick

1 cup red bell pepper, medium diced

1 cup green bell pepper, medium diced

1 cup cherry or grape tomatoes, cut in half

¼ red onion, finely chopped

⅓ cup feta cheese

⅓ cup oil-cured or Kalamata olives, pitted

2 6-ounce chicken breasts

Preheat grill.

For the vinaigrette, whisk together the vinegar, garlic, oregano, mustard, salt, and pepper in a small bowl. Still whisking, slowly add the olive oil.

Place the cucumber, peppers, tomatoes, and red onion in a large bowl. Pour the vinaigrette over the vegetables. Add the feta and olives and toss lightly. Set aside to allow the flavors to blend.

THE COFFEE LOVER'S DIET   305

Spray chicken lightly with nonstick cooking spray. Season with salt and freshly ground pepper. Grill chicken breasts for 3–5 minutes per side, until chicken is opaque in the center.

Divide salad into two shallow bowls and top with grilled chicken.

Serves 2.

CALORIES: 497 PER SERVING

ASIAN VEGGIE RICE BOWL

This easy-to-assemble bowl of fresh veggies offers a rainbow of colorful antioxidants. It calls for cucumber, carrots, and edamame, but feel free to create your own veggie combos: fresh red pepper and red cabbage, steamed bok choy and green beans, wilted kale or spinach. Dig around in your refrigerator and use whatever you have! The Asian dipping sauce can be made well in advance; the rice can be can made ahead in a rice cooker. This way, a real throw-together meal is at your fingertips to pack for a dinner-quality lunch.

FOR ASIAN VINAIGRETTE:

2 tablespoons seasoned rice wine vinegar

2 teaspoons reduced sodium soy sauce

¾ teaspoon finely chopped or pressed garlic

¾ teaspoon minced ginger (optional)

1 teaspoon toasted sesame oil

FOR RICE BOWL:

1½ cups cooked long-grain brown rice (1 cup uncooked
   rice)

1 cup shelled frozen edamame

1 cup prepackaged teriyaki tofu

½ cup chopped cucumbers

½ cup chopped carrots

2 tablespoons chopped cilantro (optional)

Prepare rice according to package instructions. (You will need 1½ cups of cooked rice for this recipe. One cup uncooked rice will yield between 2 and 3 cups, so you will have some left for later.)

Whisk together seasoned vinegar, soy sauce, garlic, ginger (if using), and sesame oil in a medium bowl. Set aside.

Steam edamame for approximately 4 minutes, until tender. Just before the edamame is cooked, drop the tofu into the steamer to warm.

To assemble, place rice, cucumbers, carrots, edamame, tofu, and cilantro (if using) in the bowl with Asian dressing. Toss thoroughly. Divide into 2 bowls and serve.

Serves 2.

CALORIES: 497 PER SERVING

SALMON WITH WHITE BEANS, ARTICHOKES, AND BLACK OLIVES

If you want to take your taste buds on a Mediterranean adventure, make this easy and delicious lunch or dinner on the fly. We love this bean medley with salmon, but it lends itself beautifully to chicken, halibut, grouper, shrimp, or tofu. Again, we like oil-cured black olives, but Kalamata work well, too, if you prefer them. Double the recipe for easy leftovers. If made for dinner, it lasts well as a top-notch take-along lunch.

1 5-ounce salmon fillet
1 teaspoon olive oil, divided

fine sea salt

freshly ground pepper

½ cup cannellini beans, drained

½ cup chicken broth

½ cup marinated artichokes from a jar, drained (3 ounces)

2 tablespoons chopped sun-dried tomatoes

1 tablespoon black olives, pitted and roughly chopped
   (about 6)

2 teaspoons good balsamic vinegar

½ teaspoon fresh chopped thyme

1½ cups fresh spinach or arugula

Prepare grill. Brush salmon with ½ teaspoon of the olive oil. Season with fine sea salt and freshly ground pepper. Grill to desired doneness.

Meanwhile, combine cannellini beans and chicken broth in a skillet over medium heat. Stir in the marinated artichokes, sun-dried tomatoes, black olives, balsamic vinegar, thyme, and remaining ½ teaspoon olive oil. Just before you are ready to serve, fold in the spinach or arugula. Toss and season to taste. Pour into a shallow pasta bowl and place grilled salmon on top.

Serves 1.

CALORIES: 525 PER SERVING

INDIAN LENTIL SOUP WITH GRILLED SHRIMP

This vibrant Indian lentil soup is an easy recipe that can be made ahead and enjoyed for lunch throughout the week. It stands tall on its own, but also complements a variety of proteins. Serve with 2.5 ounces of grilled chicken, tofu, or lamb (525 calories), or serve on top of ¾ cup prepared quinoa (483 calories). For a yummy variation, serve with a dollop of 2 percent Greek yogurt.

FOR SOUP:

1 teaspoon whole cumin seeds

1 tablespoon ghee or olive oil

1½ cups onion, peeled and coarsely chopped

1 tablespoon finely minced fresh ginger

2 teaspoons garlic, pressed or minced

1 teaspoon fine sea salt, divided

¾ teaspoon ground turmeric

⅛ teaspoon cayenne pepper

3½ cups water, divided

1 cup red lentils

1 15-ounce can diced fire-roasted tomatoes

FOR ASSEMBLY:

nonstick olive oil spray

2.5 ounces peeled shrimp

4 cups fresh spinach

¼ cup chopped fresh cilantro, plus 1 tablespoon for
  garnish

In a medium-size, heavy-bottomed pot over medium heat, toast the cumin seeds, shaking the pan frequently, until they smell fragrant, 2–3 minutes.

Add 1 tablespoon ghee or olive oil followed by the onion, ginger, garlic, ½ teaspoon salt, turmeric, cayenne, and ½ cup water. Bring to a boil over high heat and reduce to medium heat. Stirring frequently, cook until onions are soft and translucent, about 10 minutes. Add remaining 3 cups water, lentils, and fire-roasted tomatoes. Season with remaining ½ teaspoon salt.

Bring to a boil over medium heat and then reduce heat to a simmer. Partially cover and simmer until lentils are soft, about 35 minutes. Stir frequently. Thin with more water if necessary.

Before serving, prepare grill. Spray shrimp lightly with nonstick olive oil spray. Season lightly with salt and pepper. Grill shrimp for about 2 minutes per side, until opaque in the center.

Fold the spinach and ¼ cup cilantro into the soup. Season to taste with more cayenne and salt, if needed. Serve soup in a shallow bowl with grilled shrimp on top. Garnish with cilantro.

Makes 4 servings (1¼ cups per serving).

CALORIES: 525 PER SERVING

DINNERS

NOTE: For all meals, when following a weight maintenance plan, cut the recipe in half, and add that amount to the measurements that follow.

ASIAN QUINOA BOWL WITH FLANK STEAK AND KALE

We absolutely love this fast and easy weeknight fare, so much so that we often double the recipe to ensure leftovers. We recommend seeking grass-fed meat whenever possible for an added punch of omega-3s. If you're shy on time, feel free to use the ginger that comes in a squeeze tube and is found in the produce section of most grocery stores. Also, choose the Asian sesame oil that is toasted, which is not the same as plain sesame oil. The Asian sesame imparts that certain something that lures us back to this recipe time and again.

    4 ounces flank steak
    4 teaspoons Bragg liquid aminos, divided (see note)
    1 cup quinoa, preferably tri-colored if available
    ½ cup sliced onion
    1 teaspoon minced fresh ginger (or paste)
    ¼ cup plus 3 tablespoons water, divided
    1 teaspoon Asian sesame oil
    salt and pepper
    2 cups roughly chopped kale, stems removed
    drizzle of balsamic vinegar

Marinate the flank steak with 2 teaspoons of the liquid aminos for 5 minutes or up to 2 hours.

Preheat grill or grill pan to high. Meanwhile, cook quinoa according to package instructions. (You will have leftover quinoa, as you will need only ¾ cup cooked for this recipe.)

Cook flank steak for about 3 minutes per side, or until desired doneness. Remove from grill. Cut into thin slices, cover, and set aside.

In a small skillet over high heat, add onion, ginger, ¼ cup of the water, and the sesame oil, plus a pinch of salt and pepper. Bring to a boil. Reduce heat to medium and cook until onions are soft and tender, 8–10 minutes. Add the remaining 3 tablespoons water and the kale, and cook until kale is tender and liquid has evaporated, about 3 minutes. Add ¾ cup of the cooked quinoa (reserve remaining quinoa for later use). Drizzle with remaining 2 teaspoons liquid aminos and balsamic vinegar. Fold in the flank steak and any juices that are released. Mix all together and serve in a bowl.

NOTE: Think of liquid aminos as a soy-free version of soy sauce. It lends a fermented salty essence to any dish, but if you don't have it, substitute a low-sodium soy sauce or tamari. We love Bragg liquid aminos.

Serves 1.

CALORIES: 514

GAZPACHO WITH BLACK BEANS AND GRILLED CHICKEN

Gazpachos of any style are household staples for us during tomato season. We often make quadruple batches of this vibrant, tangy, crunchy soup to have on hand for our families, so this yummy chicken and gazpacho dinner makes for easy summer fare. Weeknight grilling makes life so easy, especially if your loved one can lend you a hand. (Hint!) For the tortilla, we usually use half of an avocado, but if you have homemade or store-bought guacamole, it makes a flavorful substitute.

> 1¼ cups Tomato Mango Cilantro Jalapeno smoothie
>   (½ recipe, page 272)
> 4 ounces grilled boneless, skinless chicken breast
> salt and pepper
> ⅓ cup canned black beans, drained
> cilantro sprigs for garnish
> 2 6-inch corn tortillas
> ½ small avocado

Prepare grill or grill pan. Season chicken breast lightly with salt and pepper. Grill chicken breast 3–4 minutes per side, or until opaque in the center. Remove chicken from grill. Slice chicken, cover loosely with foil, and set aside.

Place smoothie in a shallow soup bowl. Stir in the black beans. Fan chicken on top and garnish with cilantro sprigs. Warm tortillas in microwave or drag them back and forth directly on a gas flame, using tongs, until warm and slightly charred. Fork-smash the avocado on the warmed corn tortilla. Season with salt and pepper and roll up.

Serves 1.

CALORIES: 486

GRILLED SALMON WITH CUCUMBER AVOCADO SALSA

Salmon reigns as one of our favorite sources of protein, hands down. We seek wild line-caught king salmon whenever possible for its mild, buttery yet robust flavor. Although more expensive than the coho or the sockeye salmon, and, of course, pricier than the farm-raised stuff, a little wild king salmon goes a long way when you are watching your waistline!

We love the interplay between the crunchy cucumbers, fresh mint, tart lime juice, and warm, earthy cumin. This delightfully fresh combo of textures and flavors melds harmoniously with rich salmon. Feel free to substitute fresh tomatoes for the cucumbers during the summer season, for variation. If you want some heat, throw in a little chopped jalapeno for some tickle on the tongue!

1 cup quinoa

3½ ounces salmon

salt and pepper

1 cup chopped cucumbers

2 tablespoons chopped red onion

2 tablespoons chopped fresh mint

2 tablespoons lime juice

¼ teaspoon fine sea salt

¼ teaspoon ground cumin

½ cup chopped avocado (½ medium avocado)

Cook quinoa according to package instructions. (You will have leftover quinoa, as you will need only ¾ cup cooked for this recipe.)

Preheat grill or grill pan to high. Spray salmon with nonstick cooking spray and season with salt and pepper.

Combine cucumbers, red onion, mint, lime juice, salt, cumin, and avocado in a small bowl. Set aside.

Cook salmon over a very hot grill for about 3 minutes per side, or until desired doneness. Turn with a metal spatula. It tends to stick if the grill is not hot enough. Make sure to cook the fish mostly on one side, so the flesh releases itself and does not stick to the grill. Remove from grill. Serve atop quinoa and top with salsa.

Serves 1.

CALORIES: 449

GRILLED CHICKEN AND ASPARAGUS STIR-FRY

This robustly flavored, antioxidant-rich stir-fry tops the charts for a healthy weeknight dinner. In fact, it's so great that we often double the recipe in preparation for the next day's lunch. Some dishes are just made for leftovers, and this is one of them. The warm notes of ginger and garlic meld seamlessly with the sweet and salty combo of the carrot juice and the liquid aminos. Don't be deterred if you aren't a carrot juice devotee. The juice simply adds some sweetness and depth without a carroty flavor.

1 cup quinoa
4 ounces grilled chicken breast

salt and pepper

4–6 asparagus spears

2 teaspoons ghee or olive oil

½ cup sliced onion

2 teaspoons minced garlic (about 2 medium cloves)

2 teaspoons chopped ginger

⅓ cup water

½ cup carrot juice

2 teaspoons Bragg liquid aminos or low-sodium tamari

hot sauce (optional)

Prepare quinoa according to package instructions. Set aside. (You will have leftover quinoa, as you will need only ¾ cup cooked for this recipe.)

Prepare grill or grill pan. Season chicken breast lightly with salt and pepper. Grill chicken breast 3–4 minutes per side, or until opaque in the center. Grill asparagus spears. Set aside to cool slightly, then slice chicken and asparagus into bite-size pieces.

In a nonstick skillet over high heat, add ghee or olive oil. Add onion, garlic, and ginger and cook for a few minutes, stirring frequently. Add ⅓ cup water. Reduce heat to medium and cook until onions are soft and translucent, 7–10 minutes. Add carrot juice and liquid aminos or low-sodium tamari. Cook for 2–3 minutes. Stir in chopped, grilled asparagus, chicken, and quinoa.

SHORTCUTS: Purchase a roasted chicken for convenience if you aren't up to grilling. (Skinless chicken breast is the cut you want to use when dieting.) If you don't feel like chopping ginger, purchase the "ready ginger" in a squeeze tube at your local store. Keep this convenient ingredient on hand as a shortcut to yummy ginger flavor in a pinch.

NOTE: Ghee, or clarified butter, is a must in our kitchen. We keep it on hand for many reasons, mainly for its rich, nutty taste and high smoke point, but also for its range of health benefits. Ghee has a unique nutrition profile as it has no lactose or casein. Those who are lactose- or casein-sensitive can use ghee because these allergens have been naturally removed. If you've been told to stay away from dairy and butter, try experimenting with ghee made from grass-fed cows' butter.

Serves 1.

CALORIES: 500

LEMONY HALIBUT WITH WHITE BEANS, SPINACH, AND GARLIC TOAST

We love halibut for its mild flavor and flaky texture. Accompanied with wholesome white beans, tart lemon, aromatic thyme, tangy capers, and wilted spinach, it truly wows. Did you know that capers contain many phytonutrients, antioxidants, and vitamins essential for good health? This simple, clean, nutritious dinner takes less than 15 minutes to prepare and only about 10 minutes to cook. Although we adore halibut, Pacific sole, cod, or grouper all work well. If you don't love spinach, try wilted bok choy, chard, arugula, or kale as vibrant green substitutes.

6 ounces halibut

sea salt

pepper

½ cup white beans, such as Great Northern or cannellini

½ teaspoon lemon zest

1 tablespoon fresh lemon juice

1 tablespoon capers, roughly chopped

1 teaspoon chopped fresh thyme

1 teaspoon extra virgin olive oil

1 whole wheat pita bread

1 tablespoon grated Parmesan cheese

sprinkle of garlic salt

4 cups fresh spinach (3 ounces)

lemon wedge

Preheat oven to 375 degrees. Season fish with sea salt and pepper and place on a large square of foil. Fold up the sides slightly. In a small bowl, combine beans, lemon zest, lemon juice, capers, thyme, and olive oil. Season with salt and pepper, and pour over fish. Bring the edges of the foil toward the center and crimp down the middle, then crimp the two sides to seal the package. Place the foil packet on a baking sheet. Cook 8–10 minutes (depending on thickness of fish) or until fish is opaque.

While fish is cooking, slice off edges of pita pocket and open into 2 pieces. Sprinkle each side with cheese and garlic salt. Place on rack in the oven and cook for about 5–10 minutes until toasty.

In a nonstick skillet, wilt spinach over medium high heat, about 2–3 minutes, stirring frequently. Serve spinach in a shallow bowl and top with halibut, beans, and the juices. Serve with a lemon wedge and Parmesan pitas.

Serves 1.

CALORIES: 518

CHIPOTLE TURKEY BURGER WITH PINEAPPLE-SUGAR SNAP PEA SALSA

Disgruntled by the thought of a dry, tasteless turkey burger? So are we, so we set out to raise the bar. Turkey burgers can be dry and shy on flavor because turkey is so lean. To buck this trend, we added some dark meat to the mix. Then we decided to bring on the yum factor with smoked paprika and chipotle. We ratcheted up the flavor another notch with a tangy, crunchy, unexpected sugar snap pea salsa. Don't dare come complaining that these burgers are boring! Chipotle powder and smoked paprika are your secret weapons. A little warning: Chipotle powder is seriously hot and spicy. Smoked paprika is milder, with a distinct irresistible smoky flavor. Different brands offer up varying levels of heat, so experiment to find one that suits you.

½ cup uncooked brown rice

FOR SALSA:

⅓ cup finely chopped pineapple
⅓ cup diced sugar snap peas
2 teaspooons lime juice
¼ cup chopped mint

FOR BURGER:

½ cup onion, finely chopped

⅓ cup water

1 teaspoon ghee or olive oil

pinch of sea salt

5 ounces ground turkey, preferably dark and light meat

¼ teaspoon garlic powder

pinch to ⅛ teaspoon chipotle powder, according to
    heat preference

⅛ teaspoon smoked paprika

Prepare rice according to package instructions. Set aside. (You will have more than you need.)

For salsa, combine pineapple, sugar snap peas, lime juice, and mint in small bowl. Set aside.

For burger, prepare grill. Place onions in medium nonstick skillet with ⅓ cup water, ghee, and pinch of sea salt. Bring mixture to a boil. Reduce heat to medium and cook for 8–10 minutes until onions are sweet and tender. Let cool completely. Add turkey to onion mixture along with garlic powder, chipotle powder, and smoked paprika. Add a pinch of sea salt. Form into a ½-inch-thick burger. Grill burger 4–5 minutes per side. Serve over ¾ cup prepared brown rice and top with salsa.

Serves 1.

CALORIES: 509

ARUGULA SALAD WITH SMOKED TURKEY, BEETS, AND RED WINE VINAIGRETTE

If you're looking for a salad jammed with nutrition and great flavor, this one's for you. The turkey adds tasty, smoky flavor and lean protein to the mix, but it's the beets (and salad greens) that ramp up the antioxidants. Beets are the bomb when it comes to good-for-you properties. They are thought to lower blood pressure, boost stamina, fight inflammation, and detox the body. The list goes on and on, but we will stop there so you can get started on this salad, knowing that you are doing your body a wonder of good!

2 cups arugula or watercress

5 ounces smoked turkey, roughly chopped

¾ cup chopped steamed beets

¾ cup prepared quinoa (use leftover prepared quinoa from one of the other recipes if you have it)

pinch of fine sea salt

FOR VINAIGRETTE:

1 tablespoon red wine vinegar

½ teaspoon mustard

¼ teaspoon maple syrup

1 tablespoon extra virgin olive oil

pinch of fine sea salt

freshly ground pepper

Shake all the dressing ingredients in a small jar with a pinch of fine sea salt and freshly ground pepper. Alternatively, in a small bowl, whisk together the ingredients, then add a pinch of fine sea salt and freshly ground pepper.

Place the arugula or watercress, turkey, beets, quinoa, and pinch of fine sea salt in a large bowl with about half of the red wine vinaigrette. Toss, taste, and add more vinaigrette as needed.

Serves 1.

CALORIES: 516

BOB ARNOT, M.D.

THE WAR CHEST

To ensure your success, we want to cover all your bases with the Coffee Lover's Diet. Our savvy chefs introduced you to dozens of recipes, from coffee drinks to smoothies, snacks, and meals, that are simple and truly delicious. However, if you're not much of a cook, or you need some guidance when not using those recipes, we've still got you covered. Welcome to the War Chest. This is a list of basic go-to foods that won't pack on the pounds and will deliver important nutrients and taste great. These foods can serve as alternative snacks to those in our recipes (just be mindful of portion size), or combine to create no-fuss, wholesome meals. For an amazing treat, we've asked a true coffee guru to pair these foods with coffees of specific origins, to give you winning combinations of complementary flavors.

The War Chest is my personal decluttering device. While we do need a wide variety of foods in our diets to maximize our nutrition, the never-ending choices we face can lead us astray. Humans have selective appetites, so when we satisfy one appetite, there's always another waiting. That's why we can still make room for dessert after downing a big, savory meal. To combat the temptation of endless varieties of foods, the War Chest can guide you toward individual foods that accommodate weight loss, yet keep you full, satisfied, and happy. The following traits make that possible:

- **SLOWLY DIGESTIBLE**, which helps you stay full longer
- **HIGH IN FIBER**, which provides fullness and satiation
- **HIGH IN PROTEIN**, which provides satiation and energy. Proteins are measured by an amino acid score (AAS), in which one hundred indicates a complete protein.
- **LOW TO MODERATE ENERGY DENSITY**, the amount of calories per gram of food. You can eat more of foods with low energy density without consuming too many calories.
- **LOW GLUCOSE LOAD**, the measure of a food's ability to raise blood sugar. Keeping GL low is critical to controlling weight and inflammation.
- **HIGHLY ANTI-INFLAMMATORY.** Inflammation fuels fatigue, heart disease, and a host of other illnesses.
- **HIGH IN MICRONUTRIENTS**, without which we're driven to nibble throughout the day, as our bodies hunt for the nutrients they need. The chia smoothie satisfies these best.

STAPLES (PROTEINS)

SALMON

This fish is the best evening hunger killer. I buy two pieces to cook for my fiancée, my son, and myself. I sprinkle them with a Mediterranean herb crumble, a little lemon, and olive oil, and serve with quinoa and greens. They cook for only twelve minutes, they taste absolutely delicious, and I am satisfied for the entire evening. Wild Alaskan salmon is the highest-quality protein on Earth, with a chart-topping amino acid score (AAS) of 156, and the highest omega-3 levels of any fish. Lean sources of protein like this offer the best way to feel full throughout the evening. Try it yourself. One evening, eat pasta and pay attention to how much you have to eat before you feel full. The next evening, eat a thick cut of salmon. (I always ask where salmon is from. Wild Alaskan Chinook is the healthiest.) I bet you'll find you're nicely satiated with just one serving. How many servings did it take with the pasta?

TUNA

Canned tuna is a great, highly portable source of protein that can be eaten alone or combined with a quality, high-fiber, whole grain bread. Avoid tuna packed in oil, and choose, instead, pure white albacore packed in water. You may want to add olive oil or homemade mayonnaise. A half tuna sandwich made this way is a perfect preworkout snack, as well as an evening savior. Delicious and filling for hours, it will help you shut down additional munching. I recommend wild-caught Alaskan tuna. If you're pregnant, be sure to follow your doctor's advice about consuming mercury in fish. An excellent alternative: a fresh tuna fish salad from a local market. See if your local market makes fresh tuna salad and buy some for the week.

PEANUT BUTTER

Given peanut butter's high calorie and fat content, you may scratch your head about the fitness of such a product for weight loss. However, studies show good weight loss with peanut butter. A 2013 study of 262 Mexican American sixth graders, for instance, showed that the consumption of peanuts and peanut butter was associated with lower weight, improved diet, and even better cholesterol levels.[1] With peanut butter, a little goes a long way toward satisfying hunger, so be sure you don't use too much. The following five traits make peanut butter an excellent candidate for the weight loss War Chest:

- **HIGH IN FIBER**
- **HIGH IN PROTEIN**
- **HIGH IN HEALTHY FAT**: The majority of the fat is monounsaturated, like that in olive oil, and is highly satiating.
- **LOW INFLAMMATION**: Even though peanuts may be inflammatory, healthy peanut butter is slightly anti-inflammatory.
- **LOW GLUCOSE LOAD**: This is what I like best. Peanut butter's glucose load is nearly zero, so it does not affect blood sugar. This means that you won't have rebound hunger after eating a peanut butter snack.[2]

PEANUT BUTTER NEEDS A FRIEND

Peanuts are not a complete protein because they lack the essential amino acid L-methionine, but they do have high levels of the other essential amino acids. You can render peanut butter a complete protein by adding almonds, corn, wheat, rice, pasta, or other whole grains. Just adding a healthy cracker, like Mary's Gone, or a bread, like Ezekiel, therefore, gives you a complete protein and minimeal that's perfect for when you're on the road. (You can also buy peanut butters that are made into complete proteins with the addition of almonds or whey protein.)[3] Vermont Peanut Butter is a great choice.

CHICKEN

Whether you cook your own or grab a roasted chicken at the supermarket on the way home from work, having a skinless breast of chicken available is a great way to kill a fierce appetite with lean protein. For a quick, easy dinner, serve it over quinoa and greens.

TURKEY

Turkey is a terrifically satiating protein, among the lowest-fat meats, even lower in fat than chicken. With a glucose load of zero, amino acid score of 141, and only two grams of fat in 217 calories, two pieces of turkey in the evening help kill other cravings. Go for a real roasted turkey breast rather than the processed deli meat.

LENTILS

Lentils contain an amazing sixteen grams of dietary fiber in just 226 calories, perfect for making you feel full without piling on calories. With an AAS of 86,[4] they're an excellent source of protein. Along with beans and chickpeas, lentils have traits ideal for weight control and appetite suppression: They are slowly digested, high in fiber, high in protein, with modest calorie density.

QUINOA

A delicious whole grain, quinoa[5] is also a complete protein with an AAS of 106. It will keep you feeling full longer than other grains, but it does have a moderately high glucose load of eighteen, so combine it with beans or veggies to keep low the overall glucose load of your meal.

BLACK BEANS

The ideal accompaniment to coffee beans are edible beans! I've long been in love with beans as a weight-loss food because of their ultrahigh fiber levels, low glucose load, and high satiation factor. Enormously satisfying and tremendously filling, beans contain very few calories, yet are loaded with the greatest amount of fiber you can get in your diet, fifteen grams in just one cup. If you're just beginning to prepare your own coffee, learn also to prepare your own beans, as you'll derive far more health benefits and better taste than you will from commercial preparations. Black beans have an amino acid score of 103, making them a complete protein.[6] Lean hamburger, by comparison, has an AAS of only 85.

EGGS

A study[7] of overweight women found that those who ate egg breakfasts as part of their weight-loss program lost twice as much weight as women who breakfasted on bagels. Let's look at the differences. Eggs have a glucose load of two, versus nineteen for a cinnamon raisin bagel; eggs have an AAS of 132 versus 48 for a bagel. One whole egg has only 78 calories, while the bagel has 156.

OATMEAL

Oats are rich in fiber, so a single serving can help you feel full throughout the day. Just half of a cup packs 4.6 grams of resistant starch, a healthy carb that boosts metabolism and burns fat. For a perfect warm breakfast, top old-fashioned oats with fruit or toasted nuts and a drizzle of honey.

PACKAGED FOODS

Packaged foods face a pretty bad rap these days. It's true that fresh, unprocessed foods should be the core of your diet, but packaged foods do offer a few perks beyond convenience. Single servings of packaged foods that require cooking offer brilliant portion control. They limit calories, and you can't reach for seconds without realizing that, in doing so, you're reaching for another full meal. If you have to eat packaged foods now and then, here are my two favorite options for a hot lunch to fuel an evening workout:

AMY'S BURRITOS

These burritos are gluten-free, packed with fiber, and incredibly satisfying.

BLAKE'S CHICKEN POT PIE

Yes, chicken pot pies have a lot of calories, but I love these little jewels. They're loaded with chicken in a cornmeal crust, and keep me satisfied for hours.

ACCESSORIES

OLIVE OIL

A great weapon for weight loss. Ideal for enhancing the flavors in tuna fish, salads, baked salmon, and other dishes, olive oil contains the heart-healthy omega-9 fat. Aim for two tablespoons a day. Buy a high-quality extra virgin olive oil so you can really enjoy the taste. It will last you for months.

GREENS!

Kale, arugula, spinach. These are among the most nutrient-rich greens out there. Some people love the bite of kale, the peppery taste of arugula, or the velvety feel of spinach. Admittedly, though, I've never been a big fan of green veggies, which is why I love to put them in my chia smoothies. The fruit flavors take center stage, yet I get all the nutrition I know I need.

BLUEBERRIES

In our laboratory, wild Alaskan blueberries scored higher in phenols than any other fruit. Blueberries also help you feel full with an astounding 3.6 grams of fiber in just eighty-four calories.[8] They have a low glucose load of six. This top-scoring fruit provides the sweet, delicious tang in my morning smoothie.

BANANAS

I include banana in my morning smoothie because I just love the taste. If you eat bananas that are slightly green, the resistant starch in them may help boost your metabolism. They do have a higher glucose load than other fruits, so try using just a half.

WHOLE GRAINS

Despite the success of the gluten-free movement, we still need natural, whole grains in our diets. For those who aren't gluten intolerant, whole grains like wheat and oats provide greater sources of nutrients and fiber than many gluten-free foods. Pair one slice of a sprouted whole grain bread like

Ezekiel, which is available online and in the refrigerator section of many grocery stores, with peanut butter or tuna fish, and you have a filling meal that's a complete protein, high in fiber and nutrients. Alternatively, try making whole grain pastas after your workouts. Whole grains are making a comeback, as many dieters find that they need the nutrients and the carbs to feel their best.

MARY'S GONE CRACKERS

These superhealthy crackers, a blend of whole grains and seeds, are crispy and flavorful but low in calories and gluten-free. A couple of these crackers and a spoonful of organic, chunky peanut butter save me when I'm really hungry and don't want to binge.

BLUE CORN TORTILLA CHIPS

These higher-fiber chips are an ideal companion to peanut butter because they supply the missing amino acid that makes it a complete protein.

BANZA

This chickpea-based pasta is very high in protein and extremely satiating. Developed in 2013 by a pair of twenty-somethings who wanted more nutritious versions of their favorite foods, Banza quickly made it to *Time* magazine's top twenty best inventions list.

DRY CEREAL

This is a great trick if you've got some willpower. If not (you know who you are!), steer clear. A handful of dry cereal makes a tasty evening snack, with a little dose of carbs that will help you to sleep. The risk is going back for more (and more), which is why I prefer protein snacks that are difficult to overeat. Brand examples: Cheerios, GOLEAN.

PAIRINGS

Pairing foods with beverages or other foods can tremendously improve the sensory enjoyment of them. Consider classic duos that Americans have paired for years:

- Wine and cheese
- Beer and pizza
- Milk and cookies
- Cake and ice cream
- Soup and sandwich
- Burger and fries
- Peanut butter and jelly

Millions of Americans also pair their coffees with cream and sugar every day. Why? Most Americans still drink coffees with signature flavors of burnt wood or charcoal. The pairing works well because cream and sugar soften and sweeten the bitter, burnt flavors, creating a combined taste that's much more enjoyable. If you're stuck on heavy cream and burnt coffee, I understand, but I urge you to try other pairings. We'll teach you how, and your coffee will come to life in ways you can barely imagine.

Third-wave roasters, who approach coffee production and preparation as artisans, have brought about a revolution in coffee flavor. Among more than one hundred distinctive flavors depicted in the SCAA's flavor wheel are maple syrup, blackberry, dark chocolate, cinnamon, hazelnut, molasses, and honey. Pairing those flavors with matching foods will make your coffee explode with taste, giving you good reason to leave the cream and sugar behind, and begin a food adventure that will make you healthier.

How do you pair foods with coffee? It can be super simple, or very scientific. At one end of the spectrum, food scientists have begun using analytical chemistry equipment to identify specific aromas shared by various foods and beverages. Gas chromatography–mass spectrometry (GCMS) instruments depict hundreds of peaks that represent individual aromas. Comparing charts of various foods and beverages, scientists scan for matching peaks, and thus create new pairings. This field is exploding with creativity from chefs and roasters alike. You can try it yourself using a website called foodpairing.com. It's a fun site with a free trial service that allows you to plug in foods or beverages and find complements that are scientific matches.

There are simpler ways, of course. Our own noses can detect as many as ten thousand different smells, and, as you know, aroma is a major component of taste. (When we're eating and drinking, aroma is perceived by olfactory receptors in the back of the throat, not through nasal passages.) So, sip a high-quality, light- or medium-roasted coffee. As we've discussed, these have far more flavors than a burnt roast. Note the flavor components that you taste—blueberries, almonds, chocolate, caramel—and match whatever you taste with a food of similar flavor.

Easier still, just read the descriptions of coffees that are often printed on the bags, or appear on roasters' websites, or on coffeereview.com. You'll usually find a precise list of specific flavors for each coffee or blend. Then, match one of those flavors with the same flavor in a food for a simple, fun, and very effective means of creating your own pairings.

Some people like to pair coffees with foods according to roast, and others by region of origin, since coffees grown in the same areas will share characteristics. We've put together a few pairings by roast:

LIGHT ROASTS accent the fruit and floral flavors of coffee. With higher levels of CGAs, they have more zing to them, like very light carbonation. Kenyan coffees have both these fruit and floral overtones, as well as the body and taste of some medium roasts. Try light roasts with oatmeal, quinoa, or chia porridge, topped with fresh or dried berries, apples, pears, or bananas.

MEDIUM ROASTS contain the flavors we prize most highly in coffee: nuts and chocolate. Pair them with a handful of your favorite nuts for a high-protein snack, or a bit of dark chocolate, homemade granola, or yogurt dusted with cacao powder.

DARK ROASTS usually contain the flavors that, ironically, many coffee drinkers seek, yet reviewers detest: wood and charcoal. These mesh nicely with heavy cream and a dose of sugar, as we all know. Try instead a dark-roasted espresso in a frothy cappuccino for the same effect with less milk.

For more advice on pairings, I turned to a master, my friend Major Cohen, who's been a member of the Starbucks team for more than two decades. More than anyone I know, Major exudes tremendous enthusiasm for specialty coffees. Delicious enough to stand on their own, unaltered, these great coffees deliver an even better sensory experience when paired with complementary foods. A true advocate for all things coffee, Major knows how beneficial coffee can be— and how detrimental. "One thing that troubles me about the coffee business," he told me, "is [that] we sell a lot of drinks doctored up with lots of fat and sweeteners. If you get big drinks that are made with more than just coffee all the time, you get a little antioxidant, a little caffeine, maybe a lot of fat and sugar, and you might gain weight." A self-described purist, Major promotes special reserve coffees that are too good to smother with flavorings and milk products. "I wouldn't use every wine for sangria," he says. "And I wouldn't put every coffee in a multiple-ingredient concoction."

Knowing the nuances of premium coffees so well, Major excels at pairing good foods with good coffees. The combination doesn't have to be decadent to be delicious. A tiny amount of dark chocolate with an African coffee makes an amazing taste treat that won't derail your day. In most coffee shops, a glass pastry case brimming with sugar bombs stands between the customer and the coffee. But, says Major, "You don't always have to pair coffee with desserts to get a great pairing." Savory foods and healthy fruits, cheeses, and nuts also go well with many coffees.

We asked Major to have a look at our War Chest foods, and he offered the recommendations that follow for pairings by region. Although each individual coffee has a unique set of tastes, countries and geographic regions share general taste profiles that can be matched with complementary foods. Lean meats such as chicken and turkey go well with the citrus and berry flavors of East African and Latin American coffees, for example. Creating similar combinations will enhance your meals and snacks without an ounce of guilt, no cream or sugar necessary!

WAR CHEST PAIRINGS

STAPLES

Africa, particularly Kenya or Ethiopia for their lemony attributes:

- salmon
- tuna

Latin America, Guatemala or El Salvador:

- peanut butter
- chicken
- turkey

Sumatra or Asia Pacific:

- lentils
- black beans
- quinoa

Latin America, Colombia, a well-respected breakfast coffee:

- eggs
- oatmeal

PACKAGED FOODS

Asia Pacific:

Amy's burritos

Latin America:

Blake's chicken pot pie

ACCESSORIES

Africa or Latin America:

blueberries

Latin America:

blue corn chips

olive oil

Banza

smoothies (kale, chia, fruit, yogurt)

Latin America, Colombia:

whole grains like Ezekiel bread

chia

dry cereal

Asia Pacific:

bananas

Mary's Gone Crackers

We encourage you to play with pairings. Challenge yourself to find foods beyond pastries to accompany your coffee. If you discover a great pairing, share it. A quick online search will lead you to a world of coffee pairing enthusiasts, blogs, and boards. If you're feeling competitive, some roasting companies, including Starbucks, run contests for consumers who are generating inspired combinations. Now that you know a great deal about coffee, get in the game!

Coffee has come a long way from the misconceptions that shadowed it in the past. Thanks to rigorous scientific study, we know that coffee can deliver health benefits that rival many medicines. Coffee can make us happier, help us perform better physically and mentally, and increase our resistance to heart disease, stroke, cancer, diabetes, and Alzheimer's. It can reduce inflammation, and help us fight the battle against obesity that plagues our country.

To take advantage of all this potential, however, many Americans need to change the way they drink coffee, in the ways we've outlined in this book. We can choose better coffee beans that teem with healthy polyphenols, those grown on quality farms in high-altitude countries near the equator. We can choose lighter roasts that don't burn off those powerful nutrients, and that showcase coffees' natural flavors, making it easy to forgo fattening cream and sugar.

Drinking coffee in this new way can revolutionize weight loss, giving us more energy, better moods, and frequent rewards that have no fat, no sugar, almost no calories, yet a host of health benefits. Preparing coffee with manual brewing techniques will busy our hands when temptation strikes; even better, it will force us to cease the mad grab for sustenance that we Americans are famous for, and to instead slow down and enjoy.

As you put together the elements of a healthy life, I encourage you to follow the example of the long-living Ikarians. Exercise. Be as discerning in your food choices as you are in selecting and preparing your coffee. Eat more vegetables and fruits; choose whole grains and lean meats. Share these foods with your family and friends. Pair them with great coffees.

It's hard to overestimate this ancient beverage. Coffee is medicine, coffee is art, it's community, it's global development, and, of course, it's the world's greatest diet food.

ACKNOWLEDGMENTS

DAN COX AND SPENCER TURER OF COFFEE ANALYTICS, two of the most knowledgeable, enthusiastic, and inspiring coffee experts in the world.

MAJOR COHEN, who is the single most enthusiastic coffee expert I've ever met, who helped tremendously in my research for this book, especially on healthy pairings of coffee that add so much to our enjoyment of it.

HALEY NOLDE, my cowriter, whose lovely writing style has transformed this book from a scientific tome to a mesmerizing read.

BILL KAPOS AND EXCELLENT COFFEE COMPANY, for teaching me so much about high-tech roasting and for upholding a three-generations-long standard for outstanding coffee.

LISA SHARKEY, an invincible powerhouse who is making publishing great again. Lisa inspired this book and led it brilliantly to its final form.

ALIEZA SCHVIMER, the book's brilliant editor, who pulled all of the concepts of this book into a tight and cohesive manuscript.

ALAN MORELL, my agent, who has worked tirelessly to represent my books and projects with endless resourcefulness and energy.

HOWARD SCHULTZ AND HIS TEAM AT STARBUCKS, who have done so much to promote the culture of coffee, and who have given us safe and creative spaces worldwide, where so many of us can learn to treasure coffee and come up with the next great idea!

RAUL SANCHEZ, one of the finest chemists I've ever known, who tirelessly and enthusiastically conducted an enormous range of scientific tests on coffees that serve as the foundation of this book.

JASON HALLOCK, Raul's able lab assistant, who so carefully prepared thousands of samples for testing.

TOM AGAN, one of the country's leading experts in lean innovation, who helped us formulate branding ideas to educate consumers about the new benefits of coffee.

BARTH ANDERSON, for setting the standard for roasters and doing so much for coffee farmers and their families.

BILLY ANNACONE, for being such a great believer in next-generation coffees and so enthusiastically backing my efforts.

NATE AND MAGDA VAN DUSEN OF BRIO COFFEEWORKS, who took such attentive care in preparing our coffee samples for testing. Their love of coffee and passion for international development puts them among the country's finest roasters.

RUSS SCULLY, fellow surfer and best friend, for all his help in understanding coffee.

JOE BORG AND THE WONDERFUL TEAM AT ROYAL COFFEE, who sourced so many amazing beans from around the world and taught me so much about coffee.

DR. DAVID NIEMAN, for his brilliance as an exercise physiologist and researcher. Dave pioneered the mood and exercise studies that underlie this book.

DAVID MISCHOULON, M.D., who helped me enormously in understanding the inflammatory basis of depression.

MARY BARBER AND SARA WHITEFORD, for their contribution to improving the nutrition and health of an entire generation of Americans.

TABITHA AND JOSHUA KAGUNYI, for their tremendous ongoing work on behalf of the children of Kenya. They are truly inspirational.

SCOTT RAO, for setting the very highest standards for coffee roasters.

NOTES

INTRODUCTION

1. National Institutes of Health, "NIH Study Finds That Coffee Drinkers Have Lower Risk of Death," National Institutes of Health, U.S. Department of Health and Human Services News Release, May 16, 2012, https://www.nih.gov/news-events/news-releases/nih-study-finds-coffee-drinkers-have-lower-risk-death

2. Neal D. Freedman, Ph.D., et al., "Association of Coffee Drinking with Total and Cause-Specific Mortality," *The New England Journal of Medicine* 366 (May 2012): 1891–1904, http://www.nejm.org/doi/full/10.1056/NEJMoa1112010#t=article

3. Barbara E. Millen, Dr.P.H., R.D., "Report Index—2015 Advisory Report," Health .gov, January 4, 2017, http://health.gov/dietaryguidelines/2015-scientific-report

4. G. Gross et al., "Coffee Consumption and Risk of All-Cause, Cardiovascular, and Cancer Mortality in Smokers and Non-Smokers: A Dose-Response Meta-Analysis," *European Journal of Epidemiology* 31, no. 12 (December 2016): 1191–1205, doi: 10.1007/s10654-016-0202-2, https://www.ncbi.nlm.nih.gov/pubmed/27699514

5. "Chronic coffee consumption is associated with improved endothelial function in elderly subjects, providing a new connection between nutrition and vascular health"—G.Siasos, "Consumption of a Boiled Greek Type of Coffee Is Associated with Improved Endothelial Function: The Ikaria Study," *Vascular Medicine* 18, no. 2 (April 2013): 55–62, doi: 10.1177/1358863X13480258, http://www.ncbi.nlm.nih .gov/pubmed/23509088

6. Marzieh Moeenfard, Lígia Rocha, and Arminda Alves, "Quantification of Caffeoylquinic Acids in Coffee Brews by HPLC-DAD," *Journal of Analytical Methods in Chemistry* 2014, Article ID 965353 (December 2014), http://www.ncbi .nlm.nih.gov/pmc/articles/PMC4283437/

7.   F. B. Mellbye et al., "Cafestol, a Bioactive Substance in Coffee, Stimulates Insulin Secretion and Increases Glucose Uptake in Muscle Cells: Studies in Vitro," *Journal of Natural Products* 78, no. 10 (October 2015): 2447–51, doi: 10.1021/acs.jnat prod.5b00481, https://www.ncbi.nlm.nih.gov/pubmed/26465380

CHAPTER 1

1.   Neal D. Freedman, Ph.D., et al., "Association of Coffee Drinking with Total and Cause-Specific Mortality," *The New England Journal of Medicine* 366 (May 2012): 1891–1904, doi: 10.1056/NEJMoa1112010, http://www.nejm.org/doi/full/10.1056 /NEJMoa1112010#t=article

2.   World Health Organization, International Agency for Research on Cancer, "IARC Monographs Evaluate Drinking Coffee, Maté, and Very Hot Beverages," International Agency for Research on Cancer, http://www.iarc.fr/en/media-centre /pr/2016/pdfs/pr244_E.pdf

3.   T. de Paulis, "Dicinnamoylquinides in Roasted Coffee Inhibit the Human Adenosine Transporter," *European Journal of Pharmacology* 442, no. 3 (May 2002): 215–23, https://www.ncbi.nlm.nih.gov/pubmed/12065074

4.   C. Ricordi, M. Garcia-Contreras, and S. Farnetti, "Diet and Inflammation: Possible Effects on Immunity, Chronic Diseases, and Life Span," *Journal of the American College of Nutrition* 34, Suppl. 1:10–3 (2015), doi: 10.1080/07315724.2015.1080101, http://www.ncbi.nlm.nih.gov /pubmed/26400428

5.   Institute for Scientific Information on Coffee, "Coffee and Age-Related Cognitive Decline," Coffee & Health, http://coffeeandhealth.org/topic-overview/coffee-and-age -related-cognitive-decline

6.   A. B. Hodgson, R. K. Randell, and A. E. Jeukendrup, "The Metabolic and Performance Effects of Caffeine Compared to Coffee During Endurance Exercise," *PLoS One* 8, no. 4 (2013): e59561, doi: 10.1371/journal.pone.0059561, http://journals.plos .org/plosone/article?id=10.1371/journal.pone.0059561

7.   Y. Zhang et al., "Caffeine and Diuresis During Rest and Exercise: A Meta-Analysis," *Journal of Science and Medicine in Sport* 18, no. 5 (September 2015): 569–74, doi: 10.1016/j.jsams.2014.07.017, http://www.ncbi.nlm.nih.gov/pubmed/25154702

8.   Lisa N Sharwood et al., "Use of Caffeinated Substances and Risk of Crashes in Long Distance Drivers of Commercial Vehicles: Case-Control Study," *The BMJ*

346 (March 2013), doi: 10.1136/bmj.f1140, http://www.bmj.com/content/346/bmj
.f1140

9.   Y. Yamada, Y. Nakazato, and A. Ohga, "Caffeine and Mental Alertness—Part 1,"
      Coffee & Health, http://coffeeandhealth.org/topic-overvie w/caffeine-and-mental
      -alertness

10.   Y. Yamada, Y. Nakazato, and A. Ohga, "The Mode of Action of Caffeine on Cat-
      echolamine Release from Perfused Adrenal Glands of Cat," *British Journal of Phar-
      macology* 98, no. 2 (October 1989): 351–56, http://www.ncbi.nlm.nih.gov/pmc
      /articles/PMC1854738

11.   Institute for Scientific Information on Coffee, "Coffee Consumption and Coronary
      Heart Disease Risk," Coffee & Health, http://coffeeandhealth.org/topic-overview
      /coffee-consumption-and-coronary-heart-disease-risk/; Tanya Lewis, "3 to 5 Cups
      of Coffee a Day May Lower Risk of Heart Attacks," Live Science, http://www.live
      science.com/50012-coffee-heart-attack-risk.html; Donald Hensrud, M.D., "Coffee
      and Health: What Does the Research Say?" Mayo Clinic, http://www.mayoclinic.org
      /healthy-lifestyle/nutrition-and-healthy-eating/expert-answers/coffee-and-health
      /faq-20058339

12.   T. Watanabe et al., "The Blood Pressure-Lowering Effect and Safety of Choloro-
      genic Acid from Green Coffee Bean Extract in Essential Hypertension," *Clinical and
      Experimental Hypertension* 28, no. 5 (July 2006): 439–49, http://www.ncbi.nlm.nih
      .gov/pubmed/16820341

13.   Erin Coleman, R.D., L.D., "Does Caffeine Increase Your Metabolism?" Livestrong
      .com, May 22, 2015, http: //www.livestrong.com/article/460409-does-caffeine
      -increase-your-metabolism; B. Zahorska-Markiewicz, "The Thermic Effect of Caf-
      feinated and Decaffeinated Coffee Ingested with Breakfast," *Acta Physiologica Polon-
      ica* 31, no. 1 (January-February 1980): 17–20, https://www.ncbi.nlm.nih.gov/pubmed
      /7189632

14.   Ann Pietrangelo and Peggy Pletcher, M.S., R.D., L.D., C.D.E., "Diabetes by the
      Numbers: Facts, Statistics & You," Healthline, http://www.healthline.com/health
      /type-2-diabetes/statistics-infographic

15.   Meng Shengxi et al., "Roles of Chlorogenic Acid on Regulating Glucose and Lipids
      Metabolism: A Review," *Evidence-Based Complementary and Alternative Medicine*
      2013, Article ID 801457 (2013), http://www.hindawi.com/journals/ecam/2013/801457

16. Hilda E Ghadieh et al., "Chlorogenic Acid/Chromium Supplement Rescues Diet-Induced Insulin Resistance and Obesity in Mice," *Nutrition & Metabolism* 12, no. 19 (2015), doi: 10.1186/s12986-015-0014-5, https://nutritionandmetabolism.biomedcentral.com/articles/10.1186/s12986-015-0014-5

17. Meng Shengxi et al., "Roles of Chlorogenic Acid on Regulating Glucose and Lipids Metabolism: A Review," *Evidence-Based Complementary and Alternative Medicine* 2013, Article ID 801457 (2013), http://www.hindawi.com/journals/ecam/2013/801457

18. E. Koloverou et al. "The Evaluation of Inflammatory and Oxidative Stress Biomarkers on Coffee-Diabetes Association: Results from the 10-Year Follow-Up of the Attica Study (2002–2012)," *European Journal of Clinical Nutrition* 69, no. 11 (November 2015): 1220–25, doi: 10.1038/ejcn.2015.98, http://www.ncbi.nlm.nih.gov/pubmed/26130300

19. X. Jiang, D. Zhang, and W. "Coffee and Caffeine Intake and Incidence of Type 2 Diabetes Mellitus: A Meta-Analysis of Prospective Studies," *European Journal of Nutrition* 53, no. 1 (February 2014): 25–38, doi: 10.1007/s00394-013-0603-x, http://www.ncbi.nlm.nih.gov/pubmed/24150256

20. Esther Lopez-Garcia et al., "Coffee Consumption and Markers of Inflammation and Endothelial Dysfunction in Healthy and Diabetic Women," *The American Journal of Clinical Nutrition* 99 (January 2014): 172–80, http://ajcn.nutrition.org/content/84/4/888.abstract

21. American Institute for Cancer Research, "AICR'S Foods That Fight Cancer: Coffee," American Institute for Cancer Research, http://www.aicr.org/foods-that-fight-cancer/coffee.html

22. A. Wang et al., "Coffee and Cancer Risk: A Meta-Analysis of Prospective Observational Studies," *Scientific Reports* 6 (September 2016): 33711, doi: 10.1038/srep33711, https://www.ncbi.nlm.nih.gov/pubmed/27665923

23. V. Galarraga and P. Boffetta, "Coffee Drinking and Risk of Lung Cancer-A Meta-Analysis," *Cancer Epidemiology Biomarkers & Prevention* 25, no. 6 (June 2016):951–57, doi: 10.1158/1055-9965.EPI-15-0727, https://www.ncbi.nlm.nih.gov/pubmed/27021045

24. Joseph Gaugler, Ph.D., et al., "2015 Alzheimer's Disease Facts and Figures," Alzheimer's Association, https://www.alz.org/facts/downloads/facts_figures_2015.pdf

25. Bruce Goldman, "Scientists Reveal How Beta-Amyloid May Cause Alzheimer's," Stanford Medicine New Center, https://med.stanford.edu/news/all-news/2013/09/scientists-reveal-how-beta-amyloid-may-cause-alzheimers.html

26. V. Solfrizzi et al., "Coffee Consumption Habits and the Risk of Mild Cognitive Impairment: The Italian Longitudinal Study of Aging," *Journal of Alzheimer's Disease* 47, no. 4 (2015): 889–99, doi: 10.3233/JAD-150333, http://www.ncbi.nlm.nih.gov/pubmed/26401769

27. Institute for the Scientific Information on Coffee, "Coffee and Health Latest Research Highlights Role of Coffee Consumption in Prevention of Parkinson's Disease," April 11, 2014, http://coffe eandhealth.org/topic-overview/coffee-and-parkinsons-disease

28. Susanna C. Larsson, Jarmo Virtamo, and Alicja Wolk, "Coffee Consumption and Risk of Stroke in Women," *Stroke* (March 2011), http://stroke.ahajournals.org/content/early/2011/03/10/STROKEAHA.110.603787.abstract; Time, "Study: Drinking Coffee May Lower Women's Risk of Stroke," *Time,* http://healthland.time.com/2011/03/10/study-drinking-coffee-may-lower-womens-risk-of-stroke

29. R. Huxley et al., "Coffee, Decaffeinated Coffee, and Tea Consumption in Relation to Incident Type 2 Diabetes Mellitus: A Systematic Review with Meta-Analysis," *Archives of Internal Medicine* 169, no. 22 (December 2009): 2053–63, doi: 10.1001/archinternmed.2009.439

30. Matthew Cox, "DoD Health Experts Want Troops to Cut Back on Energy Drinks," Military.com, http://www.military.com/daily-news/2016/12/29/dod-health-experts-want-troops-to-cut-back-on-energy-drinks.html

31. M. C. Cornelis et al., "Coffee, CYP1A2 Genotype, and Risk of Myocardial Infarction," *JAMA* 295, no. 10 (March 2006): 1135–41, http://www.ncbi.nlm.nih.gov/pubmed/16522833

32. U.S. Food and Drug Administration, "FDA to Investigate Added Caffeine," U.S. Food and Drug Administration Consumer Updates, January 4, 2017, http://www.fda.gov/ForConsumers/ConsumerUpdates/ucm350570.htm

CHAPTER 2

1. K. O'Day, C. M. Campbell, and B. V. Popelar, "Cost-Utility Analysis of Coffee Consumption for Prevention of Chronic Disease and Cancer in the United States,"

International Society for Pharmacoeconomics and Outcomes Research, http://www
.ispor.org/research_pdfs/46/pdffiles/PCN132.pdf

2. Joanna Klein, "You Want Tastier Coffee? Freeze Beans, Then Grind," *New York Times*, June 16, 2016, https://www.nytimes.com/2016/06/17/science/coffee-freeze -beans-grind.html?_r=0

CHAPTER 3

1. S. Smrke et al., "How Does Roasting Affect the Antioxidants of a Coffee Brew? Exploring the Antioxidant Capacity of Coffee via On-Line Antioxidant Assays Coupled with Size Exclusion Chromatography," *Food & Function* 4, no. 7 (July 2013): 1082–92, doi: 10.1039/c3fo30377b, http://www.ncbi.nlm.nih.gov/pubmed/?term =melandoiden+and+roast+and+zurich

2. T. Shimamoto et al., "No Association of Coffee Consumption with Gastric Ulcer, Duodenal Ulcer, Reflux Esophagitis, and Non- Erosive Reflux Disease: A Cross-Sectional Study of 8,013 Healthy Subjects in Japan," *PLoS One* 8, no. 6 (June 2013): e65996, doi: 10.1371/journal.pone.0065996, http://www.ncbi.nlm.nih.gov /pubmed/23776588

3. W. D. Ristenpart and T. L. Kuhl, "The Design of Coffee: An Engineering Approach UC Davis Coffee Center," 2015, https://coffee center.ucdavis.edu/classes /ecm1-the-design-of-coffee/

CHAPTER 4

1. http://www.theelancollective.com

2. Jonathan Morris, "A History of Espresso in Italy and in the World," Academia.edu, http://www.academia.edu/262226/A_History_of_Espresso_in_Italy_and_in_the _World_2008_

3. Tove Nystad et al., "The Effect of Coffee Consumption on Serum Total Cholesterol in the Sami and Norwegian Populations," *Public Health Nutrition* 13, no. 11 (March 2010): 1818–25, doi: 10.1017/S1368980010000376, https://www.researchgate .net/publication/42588207_The_effect_of_coffee_consumption_on_serum_total _cholesterol_in_the_Sami_and_Norwegian_populations

4. New York Times, "Study Finds Boiled Coffee Raises Cholesterol," *New York Times*,

November 23, 1989, http://www.nytimes .com/1989/11/23/us/health-study-finds
-boiled-coffee-raises-cholesterol.html

5.   Mike Strumpf, "Keep Your Cool with Cold Brew," *The Specialty Coffee Chronicle*,
     http://www.scaa.org/chronicle/2015/07/14/keep-your-cool-with-cold-brew/

6.   Toddy, "Low Acid Coffee," Toddy, http://toddycafe.com/cold-brew/low-acid-coffee

7.   G. S. Duarte and A. Farah, "Effect of Simultaneous Consumption of Milk and Cof-
     fee on Chlorogenic Acids' Bioavailability in Humans," *Journal of Agricultural and
     Food Chemistry* 59, no. 14 (July 2011): 7925–31, doi: 10.1021/jf201906p, https://
     www.ncbi.nlm.nih.gov/pubmed/21627318

8.   Steve Rhinehart, "What Everyone Ought to Know About Iced Coffee & Cold
     Brew," Prima Coffee Equipment, https://prima -coffee.com/blog/what-everyone
     -ought-know-about-iced-coffee-cold-brew-31371

9.   Toddy, "Toddy Cold Brew Instructions and Drink Guide," Toddy, https://toddycafe
     .com/cold-brew/instruction-manual

CHAPTER 5

1.   Bennett Alan Weinberg, "Caffeine and Weight Loss," World of Caffeine, http://
     worldofcaffeine.com/caffeine-and-weight-loss

2.   Takatoshi Murase et al., "Coffee Polyphenols Suppress Diet-Induced Body Fat Ac-
     cumulation by Downregulating SREBP-1C and Related Molecules in C57BL/6J
     Mice," *The American Journal of Physiology—Endocrinology and Metabolism* 300,
     no. 1(December 2010): E122-E133, doi: 10.1152/ajpendo.00441. 2010, http://
     ajpendo.physiology.org/content/300/1/E122.short

3.   D. Icken et al., "Caffeine Intake Is Related to Successful Weight Loss Mainte-
     nance," *European Journal of Clinical Nutrition* 70 (November 2015): 532–34,
     doi:10.1038/ejcn.2015.183, http://www.nature.com/ejcn/journal/v70/n4/abs/ejcn
     2015183a.html

4.   Y. Guo et al., "Coffee Treatment Prevents the Progression of Sarcopenia in Aged
     Mice in Vivo and in Vitro," *Experimental Gerontology* 50 (February 2014): 1–8, doi:
     10.1016/j.exger.2013.11.005, http://www.ncbi.nlm.nih.gov/pubmed/24269808

5.   A. B. Hodgson, R. K. Randell, and A. E. Jeukendrup, "The Metabolic and Perfor-
     mance Effects of Caffeine Compared to Coffee During Endurance Exercise," *PLoS*

One 8, no. 4 (2013): e59561, doi:10.1371/journal.pone.0059561, http://journals.plos
.org/plosone/article?id=10.1371/journal.pone.0059561

6. American Diabetes Association, "Statistics About Diabetes," American Diabetes
    Association, http://www.diabetes.org/diabetes-basics/statistics

7. A. T. Nordestgaard, M. Thomsen, and B. G. Nordestgaard, "Coffee Intake and Risk
    of Obesity, Metabolic Syndrome and Type 2 Diabetes: A Mendelian Randomization
    Study," *International Journal of Epidemiology* 44, no. 2 (April 2015): 551–65, doi:
    10.1093/ije/dyv083, https://www.ncbi.nlm.nih.gov/pubmed/26002927

8. X. M. Liu et al., "Flavonoid Intake and All-Cause Mortality," *The American Journal
    of Clinical Nutrition* (January 2017), http://ajcn.nutrition.org/content/101/5/1012
    .full.pdf+html?sid=65b51e64–20fd-4ced-84f9–4e255a42520d

9. E. J. Dhurandhar et al., "The Effectiveness of Breakfast Recommendations on
    Weight Loss: A Randomized Controlled Trial," *The American Journal of Clinical
    Nutrition* 100, no. 2 (August 2014): 507–13, doi: 10.3945/ajcn.114.089573, https://
    www.ncbi.nlm.nih.gov/pubmed/24898236

CHAPTER 6

1. J. P. Moreno et al., "Peanut Consumption in Adolescents Is Associated with Im-
    proved Weight Status," *Nutrition Research* 33, no. 7 (July 2013): 552–56, doi:
    10.1016/j.nutres.2013.05.005, www.ncbi.nlm.nih.gov/pubmed/23827129

2. SELF Nutrition Data, "Peanut Butter, Chunk Style, Without Salt," SELF Nutrition
    Data, http://nutritiondata.self.com/facts/legumes-and-legume-products/4452/2

3. SF Gate, "What Foods Make Complete Proteins with Peanuts?" *SF Gate,* healthy
    eating.sfgate.com/foods-make-complete-proteins-peanuts-1663.html

4. SELF Nutrition Data, "Lentils, Mature Seeds, Cooked, Boiled, with Salt," SELF
    Nutrition Data, nutritiondata.self.com/facts/legumes-and-legume-products/4439/2

5. SELF Nutrition Data, "Quinoa, Cooked," SELF Nutrition Data, nutritiondata.self
    .com/facts/cereal-grains-and-pasta/10352/2

6. SELF Nutrition Data, "Beans, Black, Mature Seeds, Cooked, Boiled, Without Salt,"
    SELF Nutrition Data, http://nutritiondata.self.com/facts/legumes-and-legume-prod
    ucts/4284/2

7. Tia M. Rains et al., "A Randomized, Controlled, Crossover Trial to Assess the Acute
    Appetitive and Metabolic Effects of Sausage and Egg-Based Convenience Breakfast

Meals in Overweight Premenopausal Women," *Nutrition Journal* 14, no. 17 (February 2015), doi: 10.1186/s12937-015-0002-7, https://nutritionj.biomedcentral.com/articles/10.1186/s12937-015-0002-7; J. S. Vander Wal et al., "Egg Breakfast Enhances Weight Loss," *International Journal of Obesity* 32, no. 10 (October 2008): 1545–51, doi: 10.1038/ijo.2008.130, http://www.ncbi.nlm.nih.gov/pubmed/?term=egg+breakfasts+enhances+weight+loss

8. SELF Nutrition Data, "Blueberries, Raw," SELF Nutrition Data, nutritiondata.self.com/facts/fruits-and-fruit-juices/1851/2

3-CQA. There are several chlorogenic acids predominant in coffee: 3-, 4-, and 5-CQA are the key chlorogenic acids that our laboratory testing identified and measured in coffee.

ACRYLAMIDE. A chemical formed when substances containing carbohydrates are roasted or heated to high temperatures. The World Health Organization and the Food and Agriculture Organization of the United Nations state that "the presence of acrylamide in food is a major concern in humans based on the ability to induce cancer and heritable mutations in laboratory animals." The risk to humans has not been fully assessed and is the subject of continuing research. Limiting acrylamide intake is prudent given the concern. Acrylamide is found in coffee and the amount increases with roasting.

ADENOSINE. A neuromodulator that suppresses arousal and may make us sleepy. Caffeine works by blocking specific adenosine receptors so that we feel stimulated. Mood may improve as the activity of feel-good neurotransmitters such as serotonin increases.

CAFESTOL. A fat found in coffee that exhibits powerful anti-inflammatory properties. Cafestol exists in much higher quantities in unfiltered, boiled coffee than in filtered coffee brewed at lower temperatures.

CAFFEINE. A central nervous system stimulant and the most widely used psychoactive substance in the world. Its effects lead to improved reaction time, better concentration, alertness, and decreased drowsiness. Caffeine also improves athletic performance in both endurance and sprint events, but can be harmful if too much is consumed.

CHIA. A commercially available seed from the plant *Salvia hispanica*, which has remarkable nutritional properties. It is a complete protein, high in fiber, calcium, antioxidants, and omega-3 fatty acids. The fiber in chia absorbs large amounts of water so that it expands in the stomach, slowing the absorption of food and making dieters feel full.

CHLOROGENIC ACIDS (CGAS). The primary polyphenols found in coffee. These compounds exhibit highly antioxidant and anti-inflammatory effects, and may also slow the release of glucose into the bloodstream after a meal.

CRP (C-REACTIVE PROTEIN). A routine blood test that measures the general level of inflammation in the body. CRP is nonspecific, and can be elevated by any condition, from infection to coronary artery disease.

CUPPING. A formalized process of describing the tastes and aromas of freshly brewed coffee. This involves a professionally taught technique of deeply inhaling the coffee's aroma through the nostrils and slurping coffee to spread it across the tongue. The "cupper" then describes in great detail what he or she observes. For example, Coffee Review will rate coffees after cupping based on aroma, acidity, body, flavor, and aftertaste. The SCAA offers standard protocols for cupping to ensure accuracy.

ECF (ENDOTHELIAL CELL FUNCTION). A measure of how the body's vascular system responds to stress. ECF may be modified by beverages; arteries relax if a beverage has a positive effect and constrict if a beverage has a negative effect. Alterations in ECF precede physical changes to coronary arteries and may serve as a good predictor of future heart or blood vessel disease.

EICOSANOIDS. Signaling molecules. In this book, they refer to two sets of molecules, one that increases inflammation and another that decreases inflammation. High-phenol coffees generate more of the set that decreases inflammation.

GREEK COFFEE. This special technique for brewing coffee is used widely throughout Greece, Turkey, North Africa, and the Middle East. The combination of a powder-like grind and boiling water serves to extract the highest possible amounts of beneficial components from coffee beans. The grind used in Greek coffee is the finest of any brew. Coffee is brought to a boil, then pulled off the heat, and brought to a boil twice more. It is then poured into small, specialized cups. This is the only preparation associated with improvements in vascular function. Also known as Turkish coffee, it's best prepared by grinding beans just before brewing.

HHQ (HYDROXYHYDROQUINONE). A substance generated during the roasting of coffee that may counteract the positive effect of phenols on blood pressure. Coffee with HHQ filtered out decreases blood pressure in mild hypertensives and improves ECF.

HIGH-PHENOL COFFEE. Coffee with an extremely high amount of polyphenols in the brewed cup. High-phenol coffee has proven to be the very most beneficial coffee in studies of mood and vascular function. We term a coffee high-phenol if it has high levels of the three main CQAs as well as high total phenol content. A cup of high-phenol coffee may have more than one thousand milligrams of phenols. A low-phenol coffee may have as few as six milligrams per cup.

INFLAMMATION. Chronic inflammation is the body's reaction to poor nutrition, stress, lack of exercise, lack of sleep, and obesity. While not the root cause, chronic inflammation is the fuel that drives many illnesses, from coronary artery disease to depression.

LEAN ROAST. The very highest benefits and polyphenol levels are found in the very lightest coffee roasts. With finish temperatures as low as 382 degrees, they may also have underdeveloped flavor. We refer to these as lean roasts.

NMDA RECEPTOR. Glutamate receptors in the brain that receive N-methyl-D-aspartate, NMDA receptors may play an important role in both depression and chronic pain. Researchers have been targeting this receptor with drugs, such as ketamine, which block it and demonstrate antidepressant activity even in treatment-resistant depression.

OXIDATION. When oxygen is metabolized, the body creates free radicals. Stress, cigarette smoking, alcohol, sunlight, pollution, and poor diet may accelerate oxidation and lead to an overload of free radicals. Researchers have linked this overload of free radicals to illnesses ranging from heart disease to cancer. High-phenol coffees load the blood with antioxidants to help neutralize the effect of oxidation.

POLYPHENOLS. A type of phytochemical, polyphenols are powerful anti-inflammatory, antioxidant micronutrients linked to the prevention of a wide range of illnesses. Most prevalent in coffee, polyphenols are also found in red wine, fruits, olive oil, green tea, and vegetables. A high polyphenol intake is associated with a decrease in "all cause" death.

STALING. Chemical reactions and physical changes that lead to a perceptive negative flavor after roasting. One reaction produces chemicals that interact with oxygen, so if a bag isn't nitrogen flushed or sealed properly, early staling may occur due to oxygen and moisture in the bag. The oxidation of fats leads to a rancid taste. At the Coffee Lab, we measured seven different staling compounds and found exceedingly high levels in bags with high amounts of oxygen or in bags that were close to their expiration date.

SUPEROXIDES. These are among the most powerful free radicals, superoxides may cause cell damage. Superoxide-scavenging enzymes called superoxide dismutase neutralize superoxides.

COFFEE RESOURCES

SPECIALTY COFFEE ASSOCIATION OF AMERICA
http://www.scaa.org
NATIONAL COFFEE ASSOCIATION USA
http://www.ncausa.org
COFFEE REVIEW
http://www.coffeereview.com
THE COFFEE CHEM LAB
http://coffeechemlab.com

TOP FIVE CAFES

All of these cafes roast their own coffees and sell them online, but the extraordinary experience they offer in-shop makes each a worthy destination!

INTELLIGENTSIA: I love the Intelligentsia store in Venice, California, which pulses with excitement about coffee. In all Intelligentsia shops, in Chicago, Los Angeles, and New York, beans for each cup of coffee are measured with care, tamped down, and brewed right in front of the customer. The walls of the Venice café are adorned with bags of exotic coffees, including one from the highest farm in the world, in Bolivia. On the signature red packaging they print the name of the person who packed the bag in the country of origin. What a treat! The baristas are exceptionally knowledgeable about the coffees served in these cafes, where some of the most interesting people on the planet congregate.

DIRT COWBOY CAFE: This shop is my favorite stop in my old stomping grounds of Hanover, New Hampshire. It's the coffee bar of the future. On the wall, much like a wine list, an accounting of nearly two dozen special reserve coffees announces the unique choices you can order on the spot. A striking contrast to the many coffee shops that serve only regular and decaf, Dirt Cowboy is a coffee oasis. To speed up the pour-over process, they have a custom hot water system with spouts that allow precise amounts of water to be poured over the coffee. The beans are roasted just a few miles away, so they're always fresh.

STUMPTOWN: At Stumptown, coffee is all about pleasure, and all about the individual drinking it. What do you like? What does a certain taste remind you of? Enthusiastic baristas recommend the day's special offerings, which could hail from Africa, Indonesia, or Latin America. Headquartered in Portland, Oregon, Stumptown has shops in several cities, including New York, Los Angeles, and New Orleans. I love Thinking Cup coffee shop, which serves Stumptown near the historic Boston Commons.

DEMITASSE: A coffee lover's paradise on the West Coast, Demitasse is run by a self-described handful of coffee geeks in a handful of Los Angeles–area cafes. Each barista has a signature drink, an outcome of their love of tasting and "tinkering," which can be ordered only when its author is at the bar.

STARBUCKS LOCATIONS THAT SELL SPECIAL RESERVE COFFEES: While microroasters and third-wave roasters like Intelligentsia are famed for their special reserve coffees, the company that started it all has put tremendous efforts into providing consumers with rare, premium beans, too. When I visited their home office in Seattle, and met Major, his descriptions of coffees had me lusting for each of the amazing varietals. On Pike Street, the company's Reserve Roastery and Tasting Room is like Disneyland for coffee. It's worth the pilgrimage to experience the rare microlots they feature. Starbucks also offers special reserve coffees in nearly two thousand of their stores, in thirty countries (roughly 1,600 are in the United States and Canada, and can be found on the company's website).

TOP FIVE ONLINE ROASTERS

BARRINGTON COFFEE ROASTING COMPANY

www.barringtoncoffee.com

Co-owner Barth Anderson heads up one of the most unique roasteries on Earth, with award-winning products that often hit a 96 on Coffee Review. If you are the only person to order a specific coffee on any given day, Barrington will roast that single bag and send it to you. The roasters determine for every batch of beans both the ideal roast temperature and the best roast time. They have extensive relationships with growers around the planet and buy the finest microlots available. If they didn't sell coffee I would think they were a full-time humanitarian organization! My heart leaps when I see their packages arrive on my doorstep. I also love to visit their fantastic Boston-area shops. I could talk to the baristas all morning, and often do!

BRIO COFFEEWORKS

www.briocoffeeworks.com

This is not just my favorite local shop in Burlington, Vermont, where you can get freshly roasted coffee or growlers of cold brew; Brio runs a bustling wholesale roastery and will ship expertly sourced and roasted beans anywhere you wish. Run by Nate and his wife, Magda Van Dusen, they excel at selecting top-quality beans from growers around the world. Nate is meticulous in roasting, devoted to finding the ideal roast profile for every batch of beans, and diligent in rewarding skilled growers with sustainable practices.

KEURIG
www.keurig.com

With more than five hundred offerings, Keurig is one of the premier e-commerce sites for buying coffee. Although they are famous for the K-cup, they also sell bagged coffee. (Look at some of their ratings on coffeereview.com to find the best.)

GEORGE HOWELL COFFEE
www.georgehowellcoffee.com

One of my true coffee idols, George Howell is a font of knowledge. Visit his website and plan to stay awhile; you will learn a great deal, and you can shop some of the world's best premium coffees by roast profile, country, flavor notes, organics, direct trade, limited roasts—you name it. Here you can count on getting excellent coffees, roasted with precision, and a great education!

DR. DANGER COFFEE AND DAKTARI COFFEE
www.drdangercoffee.com
www.daktaricoffee.com

While conducting our Coffee Lab testing, we designed these test brands to see if very high-phenol coffees could pass consumer taste tests—the ultimate measure of great coffee. Dr. Danger coffees earned scores of 90, 91, and 92 from Coffee Review, while Daktari coffees won a 92, two 93s, and a 94. Both brands have among the highest polyphenol levels tested.

RECOMMENDED BEANS

Below is a list of spectacular coffee beans from around the world that exhibit the traits we've discussed to deliver healthful, delicious coffee. Generally, green beans are identified by their country of origin, followed by the region or estate where they're produced. Roasters buy green beans from wholesalers, cooperatives, and individual farms, so you can buy the same bean from different roasters, and they will taste somewhat different depending on how they were roasted. For each bean, I've listed a high-quality roaster who carries it. The list contains my top recommendations at publication time, so bear in mind that from year to year, quality and supply will shift, just as they do with particular vintages of wines.

COFFEE, ROASTER

Ethiopia Homacho	Allegro
Kenya Karogoto	Allegro
Kenya Grand Cru	Allegro
Cachajinas Guatemala Huehuetenango	Barrington Coffee Roasting Company
Gisuma Rwanda	Barrington Coffee Roasting Company
Reserve Panama Geisha Hacienda La Esmeralda	Big Shoulders Coffee
Panama La Esmeralda Bosque Geisha	Bird Rock Coffee Roasters
Sumatra Tano Batak	Bird Rock Coffee Roasters
Mexico Chiapas	Brio
Brazil Sitio Bella Vista	Brio
Ethiopia Sidama Ardi	Brio
Ethiopia Idido	Counter Culture
Colombia Huila Excelso	Daktari
Diamond Glacier •	Daktari
Kenya Gathugu	Daktari
Kenya Nyeri Mahiga	Daktari
Kenya Kii AA	Demitasse Coffee Roasters
Decaf Ethiopia Sidama Natural	Dr. Danger
Hard Core	Dr. Danger
Surgical Strike	Dr. Danger
Ethiopia Hambela	Dr. Danger
Camilina Geisha Auromar Natural	Dragonfly Coffee Roasters
Tzampetey Guatemala	George Howell Coffee
Kenya AA (K-cup)	Green Mountain Coffee
Organic Ethiopia Yirgacheffe (K-cup)	Green Mountain Coffee
SOPACDI Congo	Lexington Coffee Roasters
Costa Rica Las Lajas Red Honey	Red Rooster Coffee Roaster
Brazil Sitio Baixadao	Starbucks Reserve Roastery
Costa Rica Alberto Guardia Venecia, Natural	Temple Coffee Roasters
Guatemala San Sebastian Natural	Turning Point Coffee
Vermont Artisan Blend Medium Roast	Vermont Artisan